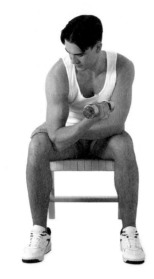

HEALTH AND HEALING
THE NATURAL WAY

SHAPING UP

Reader's
Digest

PUBLISHED BY

THE READER'S DIGEST ASSOCIATION LIMITED

LONDON NEW YORK SYDNEY MONTREAL CAPE TOWN

SHAPING UP
was created and produced by
Carroll & Brown Limited
20 Lonsdale Road, London NW6 6RD
for The Reader's Digest Association Limited, London

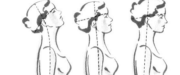

1062843

CARROLL & BROWN

Publishing Director Denis Kennedy
Art Director Chrissie Lloyd

Managing Editor Sandra Rigby
Managing Art Editor Tracy Timson

Editors Joanne Stanford, Richard Emerson,
Caroline Uzielli

Designers Sandra Brooke,
Vimit Punater, Julie Bennett

Photographers Jules Selmes, David Murray

Production Wendy Rogers, Karen Kloot

Computer Management John Clifford, Paul Stradling,
Elisa Merino

First English Edition Copyright © 1998
The Reader's Digest Association Limited,
11 Westferry Circus, Canary Wharf,
London E14 4HE

Copyright © 1998
Reader's Digest Association Far East Limited
Philippines Copyright © 1998
Reader's Digest Association Far East Limited

ISBN 0 276 42273 2

Reproduced by Colourscan, Singapore
Printing and binding: Printer Industria Gráfica S.A., Barcelona

CONSULTANTS

Malcolm Whyatt D.Phy., M.A.I.C.
Publisher and Editor, Health and Strength Magazine,
Hereford, England
Mike Fish MSc and John Orum BSc
Optimus Fitness Consultancy

MEDICAL ILLUSTRATIONS CONSULTANT

Amanda Roberts MA, MB, BChir

CONTRIBUTORS

Jane Griffin BSc (Nutrition), SRD
Nutritional and Dietetic Consultant
Professor Rozalind Gruben AHSI, RSA
Health and Fitness Consultant
Claire Hill
Medical Health Writer
Anita Kleijn BA Hons
Natural Health and Fitness Consultant

FOR THE READER'S DIGEST

Series Editor Christine Noble
Editorial Assistant Caroline Boucher

READER'S DIGEST GENERAL BOOKS

Editorial Director Cortina Butler
Art Director Nick Clark

The information in this book is for reference only;
it is not intended as a substitute for a doctor's diagnosis and care.
The editors urge anyone with continuing medical problems
or symptoms to consult a doctor.

SHAPING UP

More and more people today are choosing to take greater responsibility for their own health rather than relying on the doctor to step in with a cure when something goes wrong. We now recognise that we can influence our health by making an improvement in lifestyle – a better diet, more exercise and reduced stress. People are also becoming increasingly aware that there are other healing methods – some new, others very ancient – that can help to prevent illness or be used as a complement to orthodox medicine.

The series *Health and Healing the Natural Way* will help you to make your own health choices by giving you clear, comprehensive, straightforward and encouraging information and advice about methods of improving your health. The series explains the many different natural therapies now available – aromatherapy, herbalism, acupressure and many others – and the circumstances in which they may be of benefit when used in conjunction with conventional medicine.

Feeling at ease with yourself and your appearance can have a great influence on your health and well-being, giving you the confidence to live life to the full. *SHAPING UP* aims to help you to make the most of your body, showing how to boost your fitness and improve your physical appearance. The book looks at how some alternative therapies view body shape, providing an insight into what shape and posture can tell you about yourself and others. A good diet is crucial to keeping in shape, so the rules of healthy eating are examined, along with some ideas for cooking and snacks. Above all, exercise for muscular strength and flexibility offers a sure path to a fitter, firmer body. *SHAPING UP* gives comprehensive instructions and step-by-step illustrations for a range of exercise techniques and routines, as well as alternative exercise suggestions from t'ai chi to salsa to help you to achieve your full potential.

CONTENTS

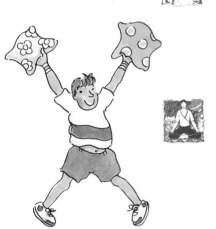

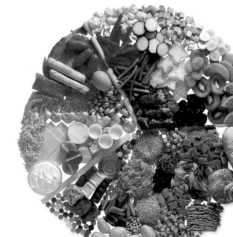

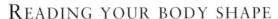

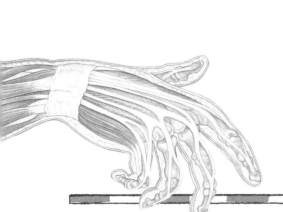

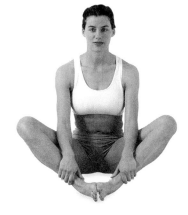

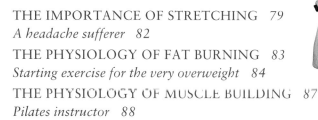

5 EXERCISES TO SHAPE UP YOUR BODY

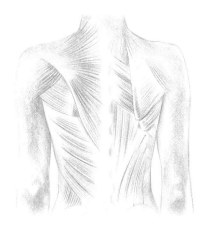

6 ALTERNATIVE SHAPING UP

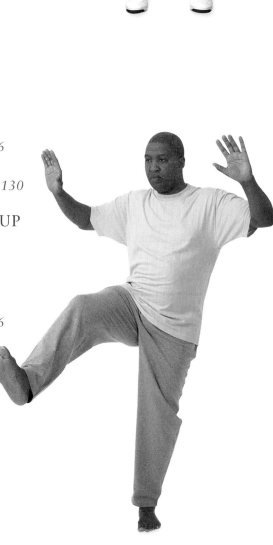

A HEALTHY SHAPE

The most effective way to approach health and fitness and achieve your best possible body shape is by combining diet, exercise and a good mental attitude.

Western society has always had an important visual relationship with the human body. From ancient art to contemporary images in magazines, art and other media, the depiction of an ideally shaped human body has been an almost constant theme – and one which has enormous psychological effects upon us as observers.

In practice, artists distort reality to reflect the prevailing concept of beauty in their own culture and society. The fact that an artist's concept of perfection was often extremely difficult or even impossible for real men and women to achieve was quite irrelevant. For example, the ancient Greek sculptor Zeuxis reputedly carved a statue of Venus using five women as models and taking the most beautiful aspect from each to create an ideal whole. In the same way, in order to create their perfect picture, contemporary advertisers manipulate images by improving tans, smoothing away wrinkles and bumps, and using flattering angles. The purpose is not high art, but the creation of an appealing image; one that will make us want to buy the product being promoted.

In recent years society's prevailing concept of perfect shape has been questioned. Increasingly common illnesses like anorexia and bulimia have made us aware of how the desire for an ideal body shape can become a dangerous obsession. Increasingly, the notion of good body shape has come to embody a much broader concept of overall good health, fitness and general well-being.

THE SEARCH FOR A PERFECT SHAPE

The ancient Greeks were the first people to develop fully and systematically the concept of the perfect form, and Greek ideals still continue to influence us today. Between 480 and 440 BC Greek artists perfected the representation of the human form, but they did not base their art purely on detailed observation of nature. Rather, Greek statues embodied the principles of mathematical proportion that were so important to the Greek culture in general. The Greeks had great faith in harmonious numbers, which they believed

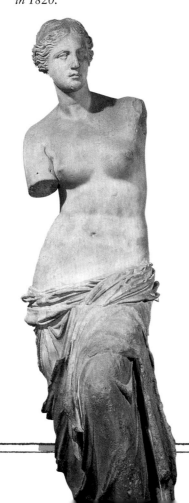

VENUS DE MILO
This marble statue from ancient Greece, dating from around 100 BC, has been a world renowned symbol of beauty since her discovery in 1820.

governed nature, including the human form. The perfect human shape should conform to a series of measurable proportions, which could be mathematically calculated. Some of these rules of proportion have survived and been passed down to us. For example, art scholars can observe in Greek sculpture that the head is the basis of proportion for the rest of the body, with a man being seven and a half heads high, and a woman, seven heads high. The measurement between a woman's breasts is one head length, from breast to navel also a head length, and this distance is equal to that of the navel to the crotch.

Another clue to Greek rules of human proportion is found in the writings of the Roman scholar Vitruvius. One of his most famous statements was that a temple should have the proportions of a man. He added that a man's body is a model of proportion because with arms and legs extended it fits into the perfect geometrical forms of the square and circle. This statement obsessed Renaissance artists, but following Vitruvius's dictates to the letter produced images showing the body looking very odd: the feet, arms and legs are overly long, and the resulting figure has more in common with the proportions of a gorilla than those of a man or a woman. This was one of the first, although certainly not the last, examples of how difficult or even impossible it is for people to measure up to ideals of proportion.

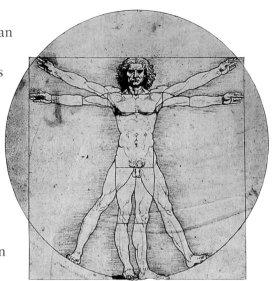

PERFECT PROPORTIONS?
Vitruvius's statement that the ideal body corresponds to geometrical shapes fascinated Renaissance artists. This drawing by Leonardo da Vinci was one of the more successful attempts to illustrate the dictum.

THE UNION OF MIND, BODY AND SPIRIT

Although shape was important to the Greeks, physical beauty meant far more than simply creating an object that pleased the eye. An ideal form represented a harmonious union of the finest aspects of the body, mind and spirit. A beautiful body represented physical strength and prowess, important characteristics in a society still affected by war and physical danger. Athletes and athletic games held a high status in society and outstanding performers were honoured for their achievements.

In perfect form the Greeks also celebrated the beauty of reason, as harmonious mathematical proportions represented by the finest physical specimens displayed the triumph of the intellect and logic. A beautiful body revealed the fundamental principles upon which Greek scholars believed the world rested.

ATHLETIC ABILITIES
Like the Greeks before us, we strive to take our bodies to the limit of their athletic capabilities with competitions such as the Olympic games.

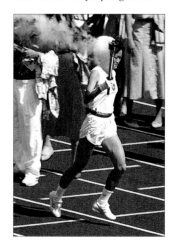

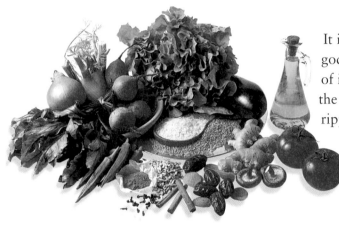

It is also significant that the Greeks chose to depict their gods, the representatives of spiritual concerns, in the form of idealised humans. Both male and female sculptures of the 5th century BC are depicted as physically powerful, with rippling muscles, broad shoulders and powerful necks. They emerge as athletes and warriors, competitors in Pan-Hellenic games. To the Greeks, perfect shape united and symbolised the harmonious interaction of mind, body and spirit.

THE KAPHA DIET
According to Ayurvedic therapy your diet should be customised in order to balance or calm your dominant dosha. The foods shown here are recommended for kapha types who put on weight easily and who should avoid too many sweet or fatty foods.

NATURAL ALIGNMENT
Young children naturally hold their spines erect and strong. Unfortunately, as we age we often lose this innate sense of body alignment. Body reading therapies can help you to regain your natural posture.

SHAPE AND WHO WE ARE

The concept of good shape signifying more than aesthetic beauty is not an exclusively Greek idea. It is reflected in many cultures and in belief systems such as Ayurvedic medicine, traditional Chinese medicine and other healing systems used by peoples all over the world.

Ayurveda means 'life knowledge' and this knowledge comes primarily from observing body shape. Ayurvedic medicine assumes a very close alliance between body type and personality, spirituality and the potential for health or disease. Ayurvedic medicine divides people into three general body types. A vata person is generally slim, quick moving and energetic, and perhaps prone to anxiety or nervous disorders. A pitta type is someone who has a medium build and colouring and who is quick to anger if provoked. Kapha describes a large-framed person, who is likely to be dark in hair and complexion and is slow to show emotions or worry. From observing a person's shape and establishing his or her dominant type, an Ayurvedic practitioner can identify behaviour or symptoms that clash with the natural type, such as a normally energetic vata type being overcome with fatigue and lethargy, and thus diagnose any health problems. The body shapes are seen as manifestations of basic energy forces that are present throughout the world and in different combinations define the personalities of individual people.

The idea that the physical body is linked with mental and spiritual health has also been adopted by modern healing systems such as Rolfing and the Alexander technique, both devised in the 20th century. These therapies incorporate the idea that your body shape reflects deeply held emotional stresses and traumas. Therapists argue that signs such as a tense or hunched posture, imbalance in the proportions of the upper and lower body, or persistent muscular pain point to deeper problems, and that improving body shape through changes in posture or massage and manipulation will help to address these issues. In Rolfing and Hellerwork the muscles and bones are massaged and manipulated to release tension and promote well-being. The Alexander technique concentrates on posture, and how to use your body with minimum effort and maximum efficiency. Many people find they gain increased self-awareness and self-confidence whilst undergoing physical therapy with these techniques.

DIET AND SHAPE

A healthy diet is a vital part of your shaping-up programme, and it is important to understand how to fuel your body correctly. Many people who want to lose weight think that reducing their food intake is the answer. In fact, it is the type of food, and not necessarily the quantity, that is the key. Introducing exercise will also help you to achieve your weight-loss goals, but again it is important to understand your body's basic energy requirements in order to ensure you remain vital, healthy and happy. Starving yourself is not the way to long-term weight control. Rather, a healthy mix of vitamin-rich fresh fruit and vegetables and complex carbohydrates will ensure your body radiates health, strength and vitality. Fruits and vegetables also provide important nutrients for your skin; for example, avocados are rich in essential fatty acids, while strawberries, oranges and raspberries can enhance your skin's natural regenerative properties.

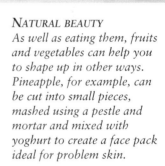

NATURAL BEAUTY
As well as eating them, fruits and vegetables can help you to shape up in other ways. Pineapple, for example, can be cut into small pieces, mashed using a pestle and mortar and mixed with yoghurt to create a face pack ideal for problem skin.

WHY SHOULD WE SHAPE UP?

Good shape is not just about looking good, it also reflects good health – physically, mentally and spiritually. As both the ancient Greeks and Ayurvedic practitioners discovered, these aspects are inextricably linked: emotional strain takes its toll on the body, just as much as physical injuries or pain do. A healthy lifestyle is one that addresses diet, exercise and issues of emotional health in recognition that there is no split between your mind and body.

Physical exercise will help to control your weight, improving the ratio of muscle to fat, and increasing your metabolic rate so that you burn calories faster. At the same time it will bring about major benefits for your general health, including enhancing

TONING THE BODY
Inches can be lost just by toning up the muscles of your body. This is particularly true of the stomach which can be tightened with specific exercises such as this oblique curl (see Chapter 5).

the efficiency of your cardiovascular system and building strength and mobility. Exercise will also improve the tone and condition of your skin as it increases blood flow and circulation. Finally, exercise has a well-documented positive effect on your moods, releasing the mood-enhancing chemicals, endorphins.

To some extent we are all limited by our genetically inherited shape: we are tall or short, large-framed or petite, have a tendency to store fat or are thin, according to our genetic inheritance and the environment in which we grew up. However, research has shown that regardless of our bone and muscle structure we can all make huge improvements to our health and well-being, and ultimately how we look, by addressing lifestyle factors within everyone's grasp.

DANCING INTO SHAPE
Not everyone relishes the idea of going to a gym to work out but luckily there are many options for toning your body. Dance is one that can be particularly enjoyable.

SHAPING UP AS PART OF YOUR LIFE

Most people are now aware of the importance of including exercise and a healthy diet in their lifestyles, but become confused or discouraged if they do not change shape as much as they would like or expect through an exercise programme. *Shaping Up* explains the specific types of exercise that will help to define muscle tone and create a more defined outline to the body. Once the underlying principles to shaping up are understood it is relatively simple to include them in your lifestyle to achieve a better, stronger body.

Chapter 1 looks at the importance of a healthy body and shape, and analyses the basic body types we conform to. It also discusses how the culture in which we were brought up, and our diet in our growing years, may influence our shape. Chapter 2 looks at Ayurveda and other body reading therapies which link shape with your emotional health. Chapter 3 examines wider lifestyle issues that contribute to the overall physical impression you create, from the kind of food you eat to learning how to get your skin in good shape, and how to choose the most flattering clothes. Chapter 4 explains in detail the principles of fat burning and muscle toning, and will help you to develop a personalised programme to achieve your goals. Chapter 5 provides a comprehensive programme of exercises that you can follow to tone, stretch and strengthen all of your muscles. Most can be easily performed in the comfort of your own home. Finally, Chapter 6 looks at different ways in which you can shape up, using ancient techniques such as yoga and t'ai chi as well as different forms of dance.

WOULD YOU BENEFIT FROM A SHAPING-UP PROGRAMME?

Even if you are not overweight and do not feel the need to restrict your diet, you may still be unfit in other ways and therefore benefit from shaping up. Statistics show that only 20 per cent of the UK population over 50 take as much exercise as fitness experts recommend. By undertaking a programme to increase your strength and muscular fitness, you may find that the benefits go far beyond uncovering a firmer, more defined body.

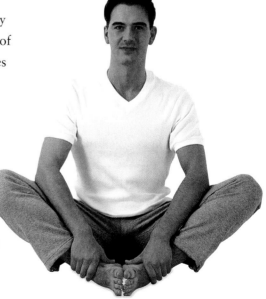

Q DO YOU WISH YOU LOOKED MORE LIKE MODELS IN MAGAZINES?

They may look stunning but many of the images that we see in magazines have been electronically altered to disguise imperfections and sometimes to make arms and legs longer and thinner. It is important to recognise that the images of popular culture are not necessarily practical or even possible to emulate. Cultural perceptions are often very difficult to challenge, but improving your shape and strength by taking proper exercise should make you feel more confident about your body. See Chapter 1.

Q DO YOUR MUSCLES AND BONES ACHE IF YOU ARE STRESSED OR TENSE?

Our body language is extremely important. Often emotional stresses that we do not consciously admit to in our everyday lives show up in our bodies. Hunched shoulders, a clenched jaw or tightly crossed legs could mask feelings of frustration, insecurity or other stress. Body therapy to unknot muscles or correct bad posture that has built up over a period of time, sometimes even years, can help to release and overcome past stresses or emotional trauma. See Chapter 2.

Q DO YOU EXERCISE REGULARLY, BUT STILL THINK YOU LOOK TOO BULKY?

Although it is essential to exercise to improve the efficiency of your cardiovascular system, many of the muscles you build up by running or playing a sport such as squash may give you bulky muscles and not improve your suppleness. It is important to include some sort of stretching in your exercise programme, to allow the muscles to lengthen and to increase your flexibility. See Chapter 4.

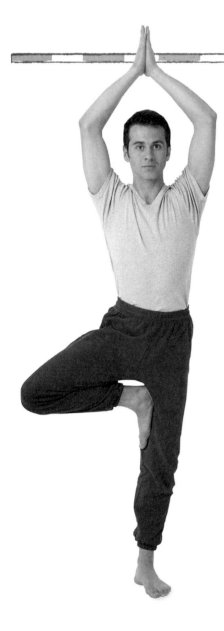

Q DO YOU FIND IT DIFFICULT TO MAKE TIME FOR EXERCISE IN YOUR LIFE?

Most people find it very difficult to make time for regular exercise in their lives. Juggling the demands of children, work and partners can be stressful, and exercise frequently ends up being neglected. However, many toning and strengthening exercises can be performed while seated at your desk working, or even while watching television. In other instances exercise can become part of your social life; for example, taking up dancing classes will give you opportunities for socialising as well as toning and shaping. Exercise can also contribute essential time for relaxation and stress relief. Many people are unaware of the extent to which yoga, for example, can build muscle tone while providing stress relief. Chapter 5 shows exercises that can be performed at home or at work, while Chapter 6 provides easy-to-follow alternative shaping-up regimes.

Q DO YOU WANT TO SHAPE UP BUT HATE THE IDEA OF WEIGHT TRAINING AND SPORT?

Playing a sport and taking regular resistance exercise with weights are extremely effective ways to shape up, but they are not the only possibilities available. There are many alternative methods that you can use to improve the flexibility and strength of your muscles and bones, from ancient regimes such as yoga and t'ai chi, to dance classes or even just walking back from the shops with bags of shopping on a regular basis instead of using the car or taking the bus. Understanding the principles of shaping up will help you to include a variety of activities in your life that will contribute to your goal. See Chapter 6.

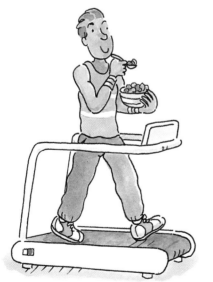

Q ARE YOU CONSTANTLY TRYING NEW DIETS BUT DO NOT SEEM TO BE ABLE TO CHANGE YOUR SHAPE?

Eating healthy low-fat food is only a small part of shaping up. Dieting will reduce the amount of fat in your body, but it will not tone up your muscles. If you do not take exercise at the same time your body may remain flabby, especially if you lose a great deal of weight. In order to tone up your shape you need to ensure that you take up some sort of exercise programme while introducing dietary change. However, change doesn't necessarily mean a reduction in the amount of food you eat: reducing high-fat foods and including more complex carbohydrates will help to control your weight while ensuring you don't go hungry. Chapter 3 provides advice on healthy eating, while Chapter 4 explains the principles of fat burning and muscle toning.

CHAPTER 1

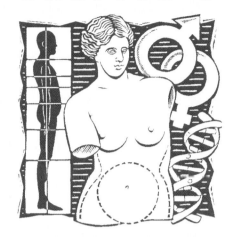

YOUR BODY SHAPE

Many factors affect the shape we are: diet and exercise, age and sex, genetic inheritance, even our emotions can influence the shape of our bodies. Successful shaping up involves not only recognising what you perhaps can and should try to change about your body, but also those aspects of your shape that you must learn to accept.

THE IMPORTANCE OF A HEALTHY SHAPE

Society's opinion of ideal body shape can veer dangerously away from that of the medical profession, so before beginning to 'shape up' ensure you know what healthy shape means for you.

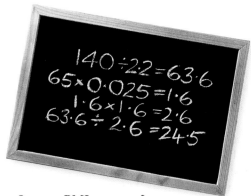

WHY EXERCISE?
Exercise is not just about increasing muscle strength or losing weight. Numerous health benefits, including reduced risk of serious conditions such as heart disease and some forms of cancer, should inspire even the most confirmed couch potato.

Modern society encourages us all to be highly shape conscious. Books, magazines and television shows all advocate a wide range of diets and exercise programmes designed to help us to achieve a slim, attractive shape. But how realistic are our expectations of being able to change our shape, and what do health experts recommend as healthy shape?

WEIGHT AND SHAPE

For dietitians and doctors, healthy shape is very much related to healthy weight. For those who are obese the evidence is clear: serious diseases such as heart disease and diabetes are far more common among the very overweight. Obesity can also result in respiratory problems such as breathlessness and asthma, as well as circulatory and blood problems such as varicose veins and anaemia. If you are overweight and also smoke or drink, losing weight can be even more crucial in reducing the likelihood of developing a more serious condition, such as heart disease. To check whether you are within the recommended weight range for your height calculate your Body Mass Index (see below).

If your BMI puts you in the overweight or obese category it is important to consult your doctor about the best course of action. He or she can advise you on how to combine dietary change and exercise to best achieve your goals, and will make sure that you don't undertake dangerous exercise that could place a sudden strain on your body.

CALCULATING YOUR BODY MASS INDEX

The Body Mass Index (BMI) was devised as a guide of what levels of body weight are medically healthy. It provides the most respected gauge of healthy weight, so check your BMI before embarking on a weight-reduction plan. You may find that your desired target weight is lower than that recommended by the medical profession. To work out your BMI:

1 *Weigh yourself in kilograms (to convert imperial into metric, divide your weight in pounds by 2.2).*

2 *Measure your height in metres (to convert from imperial to metric, multiply your height in inches by 0.025).*

3 *Square your height (multiply your height by your height).*

4 *Divide your weight by your squared height. For example:*

$$140 \div 2.2 = 63.6$$
$$65 \times 0.025 = 1.6$$
$$1.6 \times 1.6 = 2.6$$
$$63.6 \div 2.6 = 24.5$$

IS YOUR BMI HEALTHY?
A healthy BMI score is between 20 and 25. Under 20 is classed as underweight, over 25 is overweight, and over 30 is obese.

HEALTH GAINS FOR EVERYONE

Even if you are the correct weight for your height, health experts recommend regular exercise for the benefit of your general health. Exercise can improve the functioning of the cardiovascular system, making the heart pump more efficiently, and it can help to lower high blood pressure and improve cholesterol levels in the blood. Research has shown that regular exercise reduces the risk of heart attacks and strokes, and can help in the management of many diseases such as arthritis and diabetes. Regular exercise will also improve your general well-being. It is a good stress-buster and will increase your energy levels, lift your mood and promote sound sleep. Current guidelines recommend that regardless of your age you should exercise for at least 20 minutes at a level that raises your heart rate, at least three times a week.

BASIC BODY TYPES

Despite the wide variety of individual shapes and sizes, most people correspond to one of three basic body shapes. Recognising which category you fall into can help you plan a shaping-up programme that takes into account the challenges that your particular body type poses.

In the 1940s W.H. Sheldon of Harvard University was the first person to use the terms ectomorph, mesomorph and endomorph. He was primarily interested in linking body shapes and personality types. Today, however, his classifications are used mainly to identify physiological patterns and tendencies. Some fitness experts actually advise that certain types of exercise are more suitable to particular body types.

Ectomorphs

Ectomorphs are tall and thin. They tend to have long legs in proportion to their torsos and strong bone structures. These people find it hard to put on weight when young, but may tend to fill out a little with age. When they do gain weight it tends to be evenly distributed over the whole body. Usually, following a balanced diet and increasing the intake of starchy carbohydrates will ensure ectomorphs can exercise without becoming too thin. Types of exercise which might better suit ectomorphs include ballet, marathon running, cycling, aerobic dance and weight training.

Endomorphs

Endomorphs are more curvaceous and shorter than ectomorphs with a tendency to gain body fat easily, often stored around the abdomen. Their legs tend to be shorter than their torsos and they have the heaviest bone structure of the three types. A sensible diet avoiding high-fat foods is important. Types of exercise which might suit endomorphs include cycling, walking, swimming and low impact aerobics.

Mesomorphs

Mesomorphs tend to be of medium height and build with a strong and muscular frame. Their legs are about the same length as their torsos. Women of this shape tend to have hips larger than their shoulders, and gain weight first around their thighs, and then their hips and buttocks. People of this shape can put on weight easily but as they can also build muscle easily, a moderate amount of regular exercise is usually enough to keep their body shape under control. In terms of exercise mesomorphs tend towards weight training, circuit training, martial arts, skiing and racket sports.

These three basic body shapes are largely determined by genetic inheritance – you will inevitably take after the body shape of

YOUR BODY SHAPE
The three basic body shapes – endomorph (left), ectomorph (middle) and mesomorph (right) – give clues as to how your body distributes weight. This information can help you to plan a diet and exercise programme which targets your problem areas.

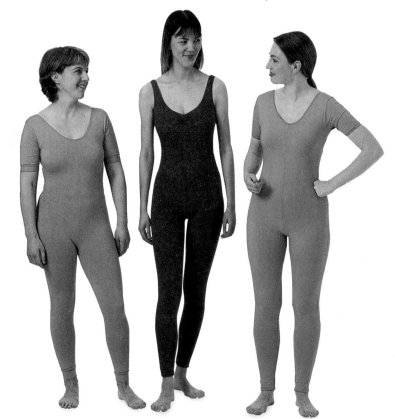

APPLE AND PEAR SHAPES

In general, people fall into two main body shapes, apple and pear, depending on how their bodies store fat. Research has shown that apple-shaped people may be more easily disposed to heart disease and cancer so it is important for them to keep their weight in check with diet and exercise. Menopausal women tend to be apple-shaped due to the hormonal changes which cause weight gain mainly in the stomach area.

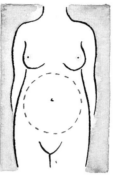
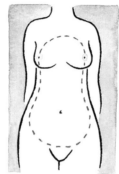

FAT DISTRIBUTION
'Apples' are round in shape and have little waist definition. Fat tends to be stored around the abdomen. 'Pears' tend to store weight around the buttocks and thighs.

ARE YOU APPLE-SHAPED?
Divide your waist measurement in inches by your hip measurement in inches. If the answer is over 0.8 you are an apple shape.

someone in your family (see page 26). There is little you can do to change your basic shape – some of us are tall and nothing we do will make us smaller. However, there is a lot you can do to improve your shape by improving your posture (see Chapter 2) and increasing overall fitness and flexibility (see Chapters 4 and 5). You can also create visual tricks with clothes to appear less tall or stocky (see Chapter 3).

POSTURE AND ALIGNMENT

Health experts agree that a healthy body shape encompasses not only weight and fat distribution, but also good posture and alignment. Manipulative therapists such as osteopaths and physiotherapists are concerned with the excess stress that poor posture can place on muscles and joints. Poor posture can be implicated in back pain, as well as neck and shoulder problems. Thera-

STEPS TOWARDS A BETTER BODY SHAPE
Many of us are unhappy with our body shape, whether we are overweight or not, and the psychological effects can result in poor self-image. Deciding that it's time for a change could be the best decision of your life, improving your health and your happiness.

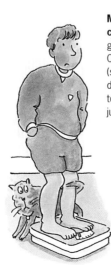

Make an informed choice about your goal before you start. Check your BMI (see page 16) to decide if you need to lose weight or just tone up

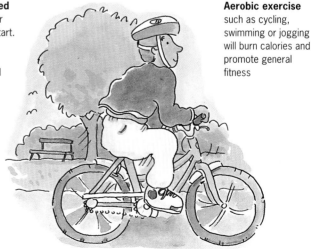

Aerobic exercise such as cycling, swimming or jogging will burn calories and promote general fitness

pists analyse how you stand and walk, looking for imbalances and misalignments in your body shape in order to help determine effective treatment.

Many body reading therapies, such as the Alexander technique with its system of movement re-education, focus on posture as the loose linchpin of good health. Practitioners believe that correct posture not only relieves muscle tension but also improves the functioning of internal organs. In addition, therapies such as Rolfing and Hellerwork release pent-up emotions.

This idea of posture and alignment being linked to emotions has been recognised by traditional Eastern approaches to health for thousands of years. The ancient Indian health system Ayurveda, for example, uses analysis of body shape as part of its diagnostic toolkit (see page 42). Practitioners believe that body shape reveals as much about general physical health as psychological states. Chapter 2 examines the concept of body reading and alignment in more detail.

ACHIEVING A HEALTHY SHAPE

Following a sensible diet, exercising regularly and paying close attention to your posture are the best ways to make the most of your shape and maintain it. Although you can do a lot to improve your posture, you may benefit from seeing a professional Alexander technique practitioner, physiotherapist or Rolfer to correct any physical misalignments. However, everyone can introduce exercise into their lives without the aid of an expert. Any form of exercise will help you to burn calories and improve your fitness, but some types of exercise will target your shaping-up goals better than others.

Aerobic exercise is any form of exercise that raises your heart rate for at least 12 minutes at a time, and will improve the efficiency of your heart and lungs. Aerobic exercise tends to burn calories more effectively than other forms of exercise and in the long term improves your general level of fitness. This allows you to exercise longer and with greater stamina. Examples of aerobic exercise are brisk walking, jogging, cycling and swimming.

Flexibility exercises, including yoga and dance, will improve your range of movement. Strength exercises tend to focus more on muscle definition and toning. A whole range of floor and weight-training exercises can improve strength and muscle tone. Chapter 5 looks at these in detail. There are many alternative forms of exercise that will tone and strengthen muscles, such as yoga, t'ai chi and dance (see Chapter 6).

Whatever exercise you choose it is important to be as informed as possible about how your body works and how you can best improve its efficiency (see Chapter 4). Reducing the amount of fat stored by your body, or building stronger, more toned muscles, is not simply a question of exercising – a healthy balanced diet is an essential component to any shaping-up programme. Reorienting your diet away from high fat foods and towards complex carbohydrates will improve your long-term health and in the short term, provide your body with the right energy source to get in shape (see Chapter 3).

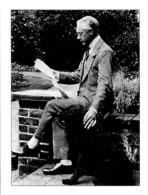

FREDERICK ALEXANDER Australian actor Frederick Alexander (1869–1955) invented his now well-known Alexander technique when he discovered that the voice loss he experienced on stage was linked to a change in his posture brought on by stage fright.

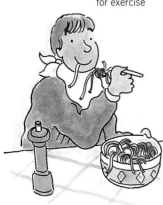

Cutting down high-fat and sugary foods and increasing complex carbohydrates will fuel your body for exercise

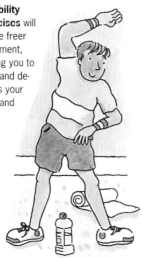

Flexibility exercises will enable freer movement, helping you to relax and de-stress your mind and body

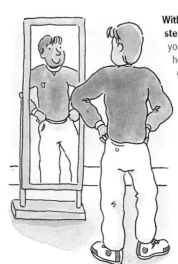

With the positive steps you have taken, you will begin to feel healthier, with more energy and increased self-confidence, just a few weeks after starting your programme

The Rolfer

Rolfing is a form of deep tissue massage which treats the body as a whole with the aim of restructuring and balancing. Within a shaping-up programme, it is useful to improve posture and gain a greater ease of movement.

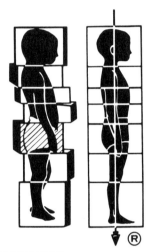

THE ROLF LINE
These pictures form the international Rolfing logo. Rolfers view the body in segments; when all these segments are balanced in relation to each other and within the force of gravity the body is properly aligned. An imaginary line can then be drawn through the balanced body – this is known as the Rolf Line.

DEEP TISSUE MASSAGE
The effects of Rolfing are cumulative. Each session concentrates on a different area of the body, working towards a specific goal. As a patient, you will generally remain passive throughout a session, but the Rolfer may occasionally ask you to make a movement, such as pushing against their hand or stretching a limb, to facilitate the deep massage.

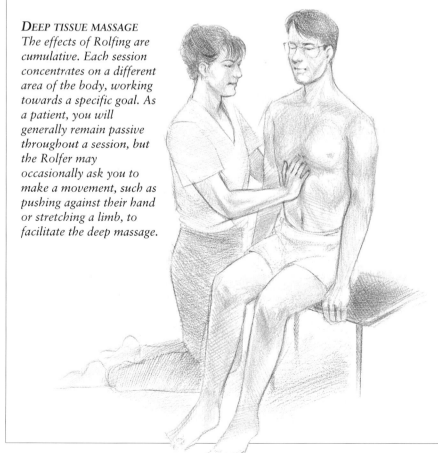

Rolfing was developed during the 1940s by American biochemist, Dr Ida Rolf. Originally known as structural integration, the technique involves the manipulation of the fascia – the web of connective tissues which surround the muscles, ligaments, tendons and internal organs of the body. Where the fascia is shortened or stuck, Rolfing works to lengthen and separate the tissues to correct any structural imbalance and achieve realignment of the body. Most people are not aware that their body has been out of balance until after it has been realigned. An example of unseen poor posture is someone who places most of their weight on their heels. This throws the body's centre of gravity backwards, so to compensate, the upper body must tilt forwards, throwing the pelvis out of alignment. The muscles and the web of fascia tissue that cover them become contracted and stressed in order to hold this false posture. Rolfing manipulates the fascia to disentangle them and allow the body to stand vertically at ease within the pull of gravity.

How can Rolfing help me?
Almost everyone has something wrong with their posture which Rolfing could improve to allow greater freedom of movement. Aches and pains caused by undue stress placed on muscles and ligaments by poor day-to-day posture can also be relieved. After a series of treatments, you should have a more upright, relaxed and centred stature. Movement should be easier and more graceful, and accompanied by increased energy and vitality and improved self-image. Rolfing can also unlock emotional traumas that may be contributing to the way you move and hold yourself.

What happens in the first session?
The Rolfer will first talk through your case history, asking details of any existing conditions (such as diabetes or heart disease), accidents, emotional traumas and any pain,

tension or discomfort you are currently experiencing. You will then be asked to undress to your underwear. The therapist will then take a 'before' picture, which will be contrasted with an 'after' photograph taken after the last session to highlight postural changes. The massage takes place either lying or sitting on a couch and will be mostly passive, although you may be asked to make a few simple movements from time to time. During the massage the Rolfer uses fingers, thumbs, hands and elbows to stretch, separate and relax the connective tissues.

How long will the treatment last?
Rolfing usually involves a series of ten sessions, spaced one to three weeks apart and each lasting between 60 and 90 minutes. Most Rolfers will allow you to have between one and three sessions to test whether Rolfing suits you. However, they stress that the benefits of Rolfing are cumulative and that in order to gain the full effect of the therapy you will need to commit yourself to the entire series. This is because the therapy is structured, so that over the ten sessions each part of the body is worked on progressively. The first three sessions concentrate on the superficial fascia or outer muscles of the body, while the next four focus on the deeper muscles or the core structure of fascia. The final three sessions involve integrating all the work so that the muscular system of the body is healed holistically.

Will I find it painful?
Because Rolfing is a deep tissue massage it can be uncomfortable or momentarily painful. However, any pain felt should be 'positive' pain characterised by the feeling of released tension which often accompanies it. The level of discomfort will depend on the individual and how much tension is being held in the body – some people experience no pain at all. Any discomfort should be bearable and,

of course, the Rolfer will stop if you request it.

What makes Rolfing different from other body manipulation such as osteopathy?
The main difference between Rolfing and other forms of body therapy is that Rolfing works the whole body rather than one specific area to treat a particular symptom. Another factor unique to total body therapies like Rolfing is that it may release locked in emotions. Rolfing can be used specifically to aid personal growth and unlock emotional pain. A psychologist may refer someone to a Rolfer for help in releasing trauma on a physical level. Rolfers believe that emotional pain and memories are not only held in the brain but also in the muscle and tissue structure of the body.

Should anyone avoid Rolfing?
Rolfing is suitable for almost anyone and there are very few

contraindications. However, it is not recommended for people with certain forms of cancer and may not be helpful for the severely obese because of difficulty in reaching the connective tissue. Recently the technique has proved very successful for repetitive strain injury (RSI). Rolfing is compatible with most forms of exercise and sports although some are contrary to its aims. For example, body building and marathon running both involve unnatural or 'bad' posture which can undo any good gained from Rolfing.

What training does a Rolfer have?
A professional Rolfer is trained by instructors based at the Rolf Institute in Boulder, Colorado, USA. Entrants must have a minimum of 'O' or 'A' level physiology and should have practised a tactile therapy, such as massage or shiatsu, as a professional for at least 200 hours. The European Rolfing Association is based in Munich, Germany.

WHAT YOU CAN DO AT HOME

A Rolfing treatment will usually involve a certain amount of work to do at home, although this will vary from person to person because individual body structure differs. Sometimes specific exercises or activities may be requested. For example, if someone has a collapsed posture at the front, regular backstroke swimming may help to open up their chest. Certain exercises which concentrate on promoting free breathing, controlled movement, increased flexibility and improved balance may be recommended to extend the benefits of Rolfing and to enhance the ongoing changes in body structure. Such techniques include Pilates therapy (see page 88), yoga and t'ai chi.

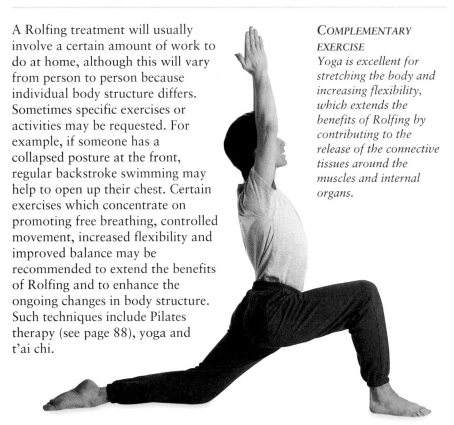

COMPLEMENTARY EXERCISE
Yoga is excellent for stretching the body and increasing flexibility, which extends the benefits of Rolfing by contributing to the release of the connective tissues around the muscles and internal organs.

FACTORS THAT AFFECT YOUR SHAPE

The shape you are depends on a range of factors apart from diet and exercise: your sex, age and genetic inheritance all influence your height, weight and build.

The most basic determining factor for your shape is your sex. Apart from the obvious differences between the body shapes of men and women, your sex hormones play a major role in dictating how you store fat and the ratio of muscle to fat in your body, affecting to some degree the ease with which you gain or lose weight.

GENDER DIFFERENCES

The male hormone testosterone stimulates bone and muscle growth, as well as male sexual development. At puberty, men experience a growth in muscle bulk and bone size. The most noticeable build-up of muscle mass is in the upper body and arms, whereas women are better developed in the leg and hip areas.

Perhaps the most significant difference between men and women in terms of shape, however, is the fact that the average man's body fat is about 10 per cent lower than a woman's. This reflects the fact that to be fertile a woman's body should carry at least 16 per cent fat to maintain proper levels of hormone production. The female hormone progesterone is one of the hormones that governs the reproductive system of women, and also causes an increase in the deposition of fat within the body. As well as developing breasts and body hair and starting menstruation, at puberty the female hormones also lead to an increase in body fat around the hips, stomach and top of the thighs. As women get older they tend to store fat on their thighs, bottom, hips and breasts as well as on the abdomen and the back of the upper arms and shoulders. Men tend to store fat around their abdomen and hips, although, like women, they can also store fat in other areas of their bodies.

The skeletal frame of men and women also differs. Men have larger and heavier bones and a narrower pelvic cavity. Relative to her height and build the average woman has narrower shoulders, a shorter ribcage and a broader pelvis than a man.

Traditionally, strength has been considered to be a major physiological difference between men and women, but the gap between the sexes has been progressively narrowing over the second half of the 20th century. Men still have an advantage in upper body strength as they have proportionally larger lungs and bigger ribcages. However, in terms of lower body muscle strength, women have drawn much closer to the abilities of men. Their performance in this area has improved dramatically over the past 50 years, while men have made only moderate gains over the same period. Currently, the best female time for running a marathon, set by Ingrid Kristiansen of

HOW THE GENDERS DIFFER IN BODY SHAPE
This young couple illustrate some of the body-shape differences between the two sexes. The female has a defined waist and hips and strong legs. The male is starting to develop muscle bulk in his upper body and arms, and has a less defined waist.

Norway, is just a matter of minutes behind the best male time of 2 hours, 6 minutes and 50 seconds, set by Belayneh Dinsanso of Ethiopia. Some experts estimate that women may even run faster marathons than men within the next 50 years. This indicates the extent to which our physical development can be influenced by social norms. Over the past few decades women have begun to explore their capacity for muscle development and previously all-male sports such as rugby and body building now have enthusiastic female participants.

Despite these areas in which women and men are drawing closer together, women still tend to experience more extensive changes to their body shape over their lifetime than men because they tend to carry more fat than their male counterparts and because of the effects of pregnancy and the menopause.

PREGNANCY

During pregnancy a large number of body changes are experienced. The body systems of the pregnant woman have large demands made of them and it is essential to rest, relax and eat sensibly. During pregnancy the calcium absorbed by the body increases to help build the baby's bones, so provided a healthy diet is followed, calcium supplements should not be necessary.

However, it is as important to exercise during pregnancy as it is at any other stage in your life. Regular walking and swimming helps to keep joints and muscles supple and can be continued right through pregnancy. Swimming has the additional benefit of supporting the body's weight which takes the strain off the back and joints. Strenuous or potentially hazardous sports, such as running, horse riding and skiing should be avoided.

Backache is a common complaint during pregnancy. This is because the ligaments and fibrous tissue that lock the joints together become more elastic due to hormonal changes. It is this change that allows the pelvis to expand during childbirth, but it also makes the joints in the body vulnerable to strain. This particularly affects the back, which is put under additional strain by having to balance a heavy load in front – the baby.

Many women gain too much weight during pregnancy and then have difficulty in

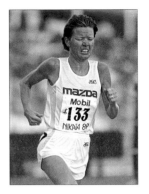

RECORD BREAKER
On April 21, 1985, at the London Marathon, Ingrid Kristiansen recorded the fastest ever marathon time for a woman: 2 hours, 21 minutes, 6 seconds. Just 14 minutes and 16 seconds behind the fastest male time, the effort was proof of the closing gap between the athletic abilities of men and women.

WOMEN AND BODY BUILDING

Traditionally a male pursuit, body building has become popular with women in the last 20 years. This is perhaps evidence of a change in the way that women perceive themselves and what society views as the ideal feminine form. The heavily muscled physiques of female body builders, with their extremely low percentage of body fat and lack of 'feminine curves', may appear asexual to some. Enthusiasts argue, however, that it reveals the freedom of women to make their own decisions about body image.

Aesthetic preferences aside, there are certain physical disadvantages for women who have such a low percentage of body fat. The production of the hormones oestrogen and progesterone, which trigger ovulation and menstruation, can cease, with possible long-term results including infertility and an increased risk of osteoporosis.

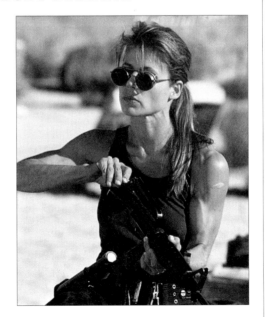

MUSCULAR ATTRACTION
In the film Terminator 2, *Linda Hamilton shows that having muscles does not necessarily diminish female attractiveness.*

Separation of the abdominal muscles

Four sets of muscles surround the abdomen, providing stability for the trunk during movement. A line of thick connective tissue joins these muscles at the midline. During pregnancy, as the baby grows, the abdominal muscles are gradually stretched and pushed apart and can separate – this separation is called diastasis recti.

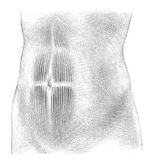

BEFORE PREGNANCY
The abdominal muscles are tightly joined by connective tissue.

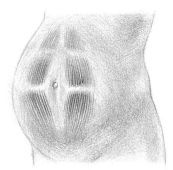

DURING PREGNANCY
The abdominal muscles are stretched apart and may separate.

losing it after the birth. During pregnancy a woman should gain roughly 10–15 kg (20–30 lb). Too much or too little may harm the baby. Also, by not putting on too much weight, it will be easier to lose after the baby has been born.

Once the baby has arrived, specific exercises will be advised by the obstetrics team to help you regain your previous body shape. However, it is also important to continue other forms of exercise such as walking and swimming once you have recovered from the birth, to maintain joint suppleness and muscle tone. You should discuss with your doctor when it is advisable to resume your usual exercise regime. Usually, in a fit and healthy mother who had no complications during or after the birth, exercise classes can start about six to eight weeks after the baby was born – but always check with your medical adviser first.

THE MENOPAUSE

A woman's monthly periods first begin to tail off and then cease altogether with the menopause. The onset of the menopause, which usually occurs during the late 40s–50s, is caused by the ovaries reducing their production of the female hormone,

oestrogen. It is this reduced level of oestrogen that causes the classic symptoms of the menopause – hot flushes, vaginal dryness, sweating, hair and skin changes, fatigue and, in some people, depression.

Lack of oestrogen also slows the body's metabolic rate (the rate at which the body uses energy to fuel all physiological functions) but this may not manifest itself until later. Metabolic changes include an increase in the level of fats in the blood, which increases the likelihood of a narrowing of the arteries (atherosclerosis) and also the chances of coronary artery disease and a stroke.

The effect the menopause has on bones is one of the most damaging changes. During the first two to five years of the menopause, the bones become thinner. Over a period of 10 to 15 years from the onset of the menopause, osteoporosis (an increase in the brittleness of the bones) may develop.

Slight weight gain may be experienced, due in part to the slowing of the metabolism, but also because as we age we tend to exercise less. A more obvious change that takes place around menopause is the change in how fat is distributed within the body. Before menopause fat is typically distributed

---

CORRECTING SEPARATION OF THE ABDOMINAL MUSCLES

Separation of the abdominal muscles happens when the muscles can stretch no further and may not be noticeable during your first pregnancy. Here we show how to check for separation and how to

repair the split. The correction exercise should be performed for ten repetitions at least five times a day. After a week or two, the gap should return to normal – about 1.25 cm (½ in).

CHECKING FOR SEPARATION
Lie on your back with knees bent and feel down the midline of your abdomen for the gap in between your abdominal muscles. If you can fit more than two fingers in the gap, your muscles have separated.

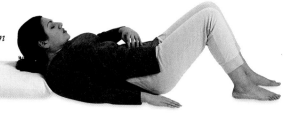

CORRECTING THE SEPARATION
Take a deep breath and, as you exhale, lift your head up; after a few days, you should be able to lift your shoulders too. At the same time, gently pull the two sides of the abdominal muscles towards the midline of your stomach. Lie back slowly and repeat.

OSTEOPOROSIS AND BODY SHAPE

With age, body shape can sometimes change due to the effects of the brittle-bone condition osteoporosis. In its severe form the condition causes curvature of the spine, or 'dowager's hump'; as well as a general loss of height. Osteoporosis is a progressive loss of bone density which, over time, results in the bones becoming brittle and easily broken. The vertebrae in the spine may crumble, causing the spine to compress and curve forwards. Mild osteoporosis is a natural part of ageing, but the severe form, which is more common in women, can be crippling. Preventive steps include a calcium-rich diet, regular exercise throughout life, and hormone replacement therapy for postmenopausal women.

BONE DENSITY
In healthy bone (below) fibres of the protein collagen provide density and elasticity while calcium gives hardness. In osteoporitic bone (right), loss of calcium causes brittleness which leads to fractures, and spinal curvature (right).

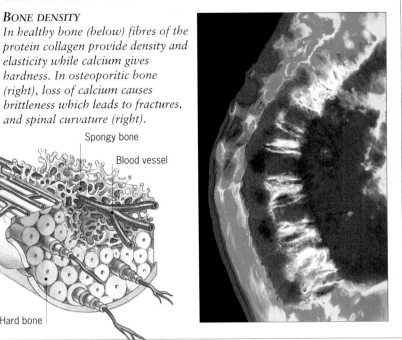

Spongy bone

Blood vessel

Hard bone

around the buttocks and thighs, as well as the stomach. After menopause, however, a larger proportion of fat tends to be stored around the front of the stomach and around the abdomen.

All of these body changes are normal, but their effects can be minimised by adjusting your lifestyle to include the right type of exercise programme. Remember, the earlier you start, the more chance you have of lessening the effects of the menopause.

Weight-bearing exercises strengthen both the bones and the muscles, while aerobic exercise strengthens the heart and the lungs.

Diet is also important. Before the age of 35 years bones are still growing, so a diet that includes enough calcium, and vitamin D to metabolise the calcium, will help to provide you with stronger bones. If you are over 35 years, it is still important to take in enough calcium as this will slow down the rate at which bone mass is lost. Some dietary experts advise an intake of at least 1000 mg of calcium per day for pre and postmenopausal women.

AGEING AND BODY SHAPE

The ageing process has clear effects on the shape of our bodies, although many changes are not inevitable and are as much a result of changes in activities and a more sedentary lifestyle as the ageing process itself.

Weight gain seems to be a common feature of ageing. Metabolism slows down with age making it more difficult to lose weight. After the age of 30 your metabolic rate declines by approximately 2 per cent each decade. The ratio of muscle to fat also alters with age with a shift in favour of fat. However, the effects of all these changes can be slowed with regular exercise. Recent evidence suggests that the most influential factor in the age-related shape changes is the fact that people become more sedentary as they get older.

Many people also see frailty and loss of muscle strength as an inevitable effect of ageing, but, recent research examining the extent to which the elderly can improve their muscle strength through exercise has shown that huge improvements can be made even in old age (see right).

GENETIC INHERITANCE AND ENVIRONMENTAL INFLUENCES

Your body shape is very much dictated by what your parents look like, what your grandparents looked like and, sometimes, what an ancient ancestor looked like. This programming is carried in your genes.

Certain predominant characteristics are handed down through our family trees. Our height, shape and even weight are influenced by our genetic inheritance. Genes are

STRENGTH IN OLD AGE
A study in 1990 by Dr Maria Fiatarone in the United States showed how exercise can improve quality of life in old age. After eight weeks of weight training, 10 men and women aged from 87 to 96 almost tripled their muscle strength and found they could get around much easier. Their confidence soared – one man said he felt 50 again.

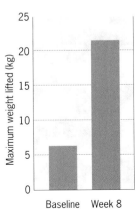

25

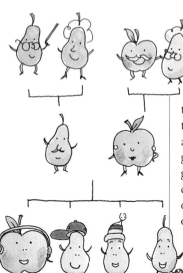

FAMILY TREE OF
BODY SHAPE
A person's height and
build are believed to be
controlled by the
combined effects of many
genes, along with
environmental effects
such as upbringing, diet
and exercise. The family
tree shown here consists
of apple and pear-shaped
people. A child's
tendency towards a
certain shape depends on
the relative number of
body-shape determining
genes handed down from
the parents.

contained in chromosomes within a person's body cells. Each chromosome contains a long strand of the hereditary substance deoxyribonucleic acid, or DNA, which transmits genetic information. When two short people have a child there is a high chance that the child will also be short as he or she will inherit the genetic tendency to be 'short' from the genetic pools of both parents. However, quantitative characteristics, such as height or skin colour are controlled by a number of different genetic instructions which interact in complex ways. This is known as 'polygenic inheritance' and makes it difficult to identify a simple pattern of dominant or recessive traits. It is possible, for example, that two short people might produce a very tall child, depending on the interaction of different commands in the genetic blueprint.

Environmental factors such as the quality of healthcare and nutrition enjoyed by a child can also influence adult height, although maximum potential size might be genetically 'capped' at a certain level. Research has shown that as diet improves children gain in height regardless of their inheritance. The height gains measured in postwar children in Britain have widely been attributed to the introduction of nutritionally balanced school dinners during the Second World War. Increased intakes of calcium have been shown to be particularly important in this regard. The amount of regular exercise performed during childhood and adolescence also plays a role in encouraging the healthy growth of organs, bones and muscles. The size of your lungs is largely determined by the level of aerobic exercise that you performed during adolescence when your lungs were still developing.

GENES AND HOW THEY AFFECT YOUR SHAPE

Genes are units of hereditary material that are contained in the body's cells. They help to determine all aspects of bodily growth and functioning by directing the manufacture of proteins. All of a person's genes come directly from their parents. The genes are contained in a chain of deoxyribonucleic acid, or DNA, which makes up each of the 46 chromosomes that are held in every body cell. Each body cell houses this identical structure, or DNA. Everyone has a different DNA pattern making us all distinct individuals with different eye and hair colour, body shape, physical and behavioural characteristics. The only individuals to share the same DNA are identical twins.

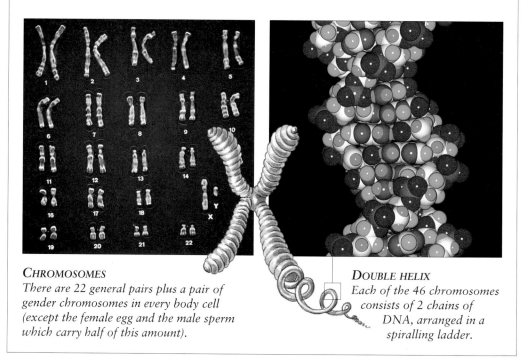

CHROMOSOMES
There are 22 general pairs plus a pair of
gender chromosomes in every body cell
(except the female egg and the male sperm
which carry half of this amount).

DOUBLE HELIX
Each of the 46 chromosomes
consists of 2 chains of
DNA, arranged in a
spiralling ladder.

FAMILY RESEMBLANCE

Visual characteristics can be passed from one generation to the next, or perhaps skip a generation, only to reappear later. One famous example is the Habsburg lip. The Habsburg dynasty flourished from the 15th to the 19th century and intermarriage with the royal houses of Europe produced the striking family trait of a very prominent lower lip. It can be seen in many family portraits. Examples of family resemblances are also evident in the generations of the British royal family. Intermarriage with other royal families, such as the Romanovs of Russia in the 19th century, has led to some recurring resemblances.

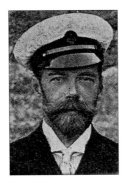
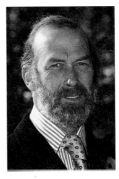

ROYAL LIKENESS
Blood relatives through the female line, Britain's Prince Michael of Kent (right) and Tsar Nicholas II of Russia (left) share family characteristics passed down for centuries.

BODY SHAPE AND RACE

There is a noticeable difference in body shapes between different races. Anthropologists have many theories about how these various body shapes evolved. Their research has shown that there is a relationship between a people's average shape and weight and the climate that they inhabit.

The colder the temperature, the more body fat people tend to carry. A rounded, short-limbed body shape conserves heat more efficiently, and this body shape is predominant in the Arctic regions.

The most efficient way to lose heat from the body is to have an extended surface area from which to lose it and accordingly desert-living peoples such as the Australian aborigines and many African tribes have long, slender arms and legs.

Body shape is also governed by the diet available to live on. Anthropologists believe that the body shape of peoples living in poorly nourished countries gradually changed in order to ensure their survival. In an area ranging from Egypt to India, southern China and South-east Asia, a body shape developed that was small and slight. This was because the smaller the body, the fewer calories it required for survival. As the body shape of people living in this wide area became progressively smaller, it meant that they could produce more and more work on a smaller and smaller intake of calories. In contrast, countries such as Australia and New Zealand have tall populations. This is partly because of intermarriage between different types of peoples, but the increased height of people who are from a traditionally short Celtic-Irish background has been attributed to the high protein and high calcium diet typical of these countries.

Very many variations on these broad principles occur, governed by the human's ability to modify diet and the environment by growing and rearing food and by building shelters as protection from the elements. This talent enables people of the 'wrong' shape to live successfully in 'hostile' environments.

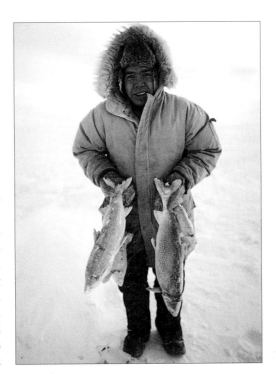

KEEPING WARM IN THE ARCTIC
Indigenous to the Arctic region, the Inuit are a good example of how human body shape adapts to the environment. Their characteristically short and squat body shape conserves energy efficiently. Traditionally, the Inuit wore animal skins to keep themselves warm. Today, however, modern clothing such as Gortex and Polartec keep out the elements – and help visitors from other climates to also keep warm.

Perceptions of 'Normal' Shape

Before beginning a shaping-up programme it may be helpful to think about how much your ideal shape is influenced by the often unrealistic dictates of fashion and society.

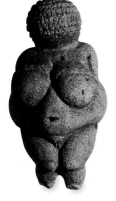

VENUS OF WILLENDORF
This ancient sandstone sculpture dates from the Palaeolithic period, around 20 000 BC. The very full figure celebrates the beauty of the fertile female form.

SHAPE AND POWER
The wealth and status of King Henry VIII was conveyed by his imposing figure. At a time when malnutrition posed a real threat to large numbers of ordinary people, Henry continued to gain weight, symbolising his own personal prosperity throughout his reign.

Throughout the ages the 'acceptable' shape of women, and to a far lesser degree men, has varied – and people have always responded to the fashions of their day. The chances of your natural body shape being fashionable are quite random and yet people will go to great lengths to try to achieve a body shape that contradicts their genetic inheritance if that is what fashion demands.

CHANGES THROUGH HISTORY

Although today Western society associates attractiveness with being slim, thin has not always been in fashion. From ancient cultures up until the 19th century, fat has been associated with a woman's fertility, and up until the latter part of the 20th century fertility was greatly valued. Neolithic fertility goddesses were round-bellied, wide-hipped

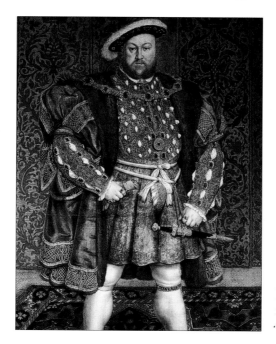

and full-breasted, reflecting the ideal woman to ensure a man's genetic line. The worship of mother figures continued with the adoration of the Madonna, Renaissance paintings of the Virgin focusing on the breasts and belly, without actually depicting any flesh: her modesty was protected with generous swathes of cloth.

Fat was not solely associated with women and fertility; it also indicated a person's wealth and status. The rich could afford to eat more and were less likely to perform physical activity. Similarly the courtesans of the courts of Europe for much of the past three centuries were large, plump women: lazy, indolent and given over to hedonism.

For men, there has been pressure throughout the centuries to present a manly figure. Doublet and hose revealed quite an expanse of male leg from the 14th century onwards, hemlines rising so high that by the mid 15th century modesty dictated the need for a codpiece. Occasionally men used padding and binding to improve on nature. It was not uncommon for 18th-century beaux to use padding on their calves.

However, while being thin may only relatively recently have become fashionable, manipulating shapes to exaggerate the narrowness of a woman's waist in relation to her bust and hips has had a long tradition. Some theorists argue this is because men are genetically programmed to associate a good waist/hip ratio with fertility: in the interests of protecting their genetic line they have an 'eye' for childbearing hips indicated by a slim waist. To achieve this, corsetry was used for centuries: in the Victorian and Edwardian eras a tiny waist was accompanied by first crinolines and then the bustle ·to exaggerate the hips and bottom. Such a

FASHION AND 'IDEAL' BODY SHAPE

Today's fashion industry is often blamed for contributing to the rise of eating disorders such as anorexia and bulimia nervosa as people strive to be thinner and 'sexier'. However, fashion has dictated body shape and defined sexuality for many centuries.

So-called 'ideal' shape has always had a powerful effect. Some Edwardian women, for example, had their lower ribs surgically removed so that their corsets could be pulled tighter to achieve the hourglass figure that was fashionable at the time.

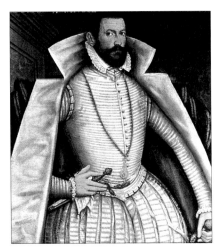

ELIZABETHAN ELAN
Elizabethan men were as figure conscious as women. Corsets were used to reduce their waists, with pantaloons exaggerating the effects.

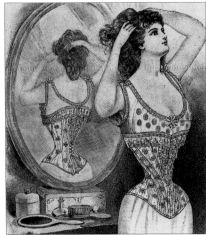

EDWARDIAN CORSETRY
Edwardian fashion demanded impossibly petite waists achievable only with heavy corsetry that distorted the spine and compressed the stomach.

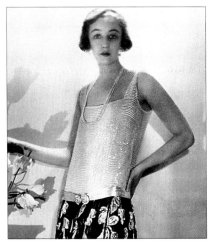

1920S MINIMALISM
Fashionable body shape for women in the 1920s was slim, boyish and sporty. Clothes skimmed waists and breasts were bound to achieve a flat chest.

physique was so unnatural that it could only be achieved with the aid of tightly laced corsets. Such was the appeal of this fashion, that some Edwardian men also adopted corsets to achieve a slimmer waist. For both women and men, tight lacing dangerously compressed the abdominal organs and made breathing laboured. Exercise was uncomfortable, but then, only the most moderate of exertion was considered genteel.

At the end of the First World War when women got the vote, their new freedom was reflected in their dress. The 'flapper' look allowed free movement and skirts rose daringly to the knee, revealing women's legs for the first time in history. The fashionable body shape of the time was flat-chested and sporty, so women began dieting for the first time and binding their breasts to make them look smaller. In the young upper class set, it became fashionable to take drugs to achieve a slim figure, a trend which has continued throughout the following decades.

After the Second World War there was initially a widespread push towards a return to traditional values. Women were encouraged by government policy to leave the workforce and return to their traditional role as homemaker and mother. Welfare schemes were aimed at allowing women to remain at home while their husbands worked to support the family. Christian Dior's 'New Look' in many ways emphasised a womanly figure, with full skirts exaggerating the width of the hips, and breasts pushed forward in very structured conical-shaped bras. Nipped waistlines exaggerated curves further still. The traditional male role as provider and protector was emphasised by wide-shouldered suits giving an impression of strength and power.

Another revolution occurred in the 1960s with the arrival of the mini skirt. It was during this period that female attractiveness became firmly linked with youth. Motherhood was out of fashion: society was inspired by the culture of youth and models like Twiggy set a new vogue for thin, boyish figures. Designers followed suit with shapeless shift dresses disguising natural female curves. Fashion for men also started to focus on boyish shapes: the Mod look, with

SYMPTOMS OF ANOREXIA

There are a number of behavioural and physical indicators that suggest anorexia. These are:

► *Rapid and very noticeable weight loss – ranging from 25 per cent to 33 per cent of the sufferer's normal weight.*

► *Hyperactivity.*

► *Obsessive exercising.*

► *Preoccupation with food.*

► *Unwillingness to eat in company.*

► *Hiding food.*

► *Inability to sleep.*

► *Disruption or cessation of menstrual cycle.*

► *An increase in the density of the soft coating of hair covering the skin.*

its drainpipe jeans and tight-fitting shirts, was designed for the thin boyish figure of popstars such as Roger Daltry.

Although today we may think we have a more balanced view about appearance, there is still plenty of evidence that we will go to often extreme lengths to achieve an ideal shape. Slimness is still the order of the day, but with the added pressure on women to have curves in the 'right' places. Eating disorders appear to be increasing among both sexes, while cosmetic surgery has recently become a popular option for both men and women unhappy with their shape. Although there are surgical options for changing body shape, any decision to undergo surgery should be well researched and thought through.

DISTORTED SHAPE PERCEPTION

At some stage we all would like to change aspects of our shape, but for some people shape becomes a dangerous obsession. A lack of self-confidence and self-esteem can lead to focusing on shape as the solution to a person's unhappiness. In extreme cases the eating disorders anorexia and bulimia can develop as a result. These illnesses are psychologically based and cause severe physical problems. Sufferers have a terror of putting on weight and have a very distorted view of their bodies – even at their most gaunt they believe they are fat and ugly. Such a negative self-image and a striving for an unrealistic body shape causes such distress that

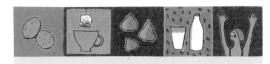

SUPER SHAPER

It is a myth that potatoes are fattening. In fact, they are mostly carbohydrate which is an energy food with only half the calories of fat. It is the oil or fat that is used to cook potatoes, or added as a topping, that makes them fattening. Potatoes also contain protein and fibre and are good sources of potassium and vitamin C. For healthy eating, avoid fried potatoes and crisps and opt for boiled or baked potatoes. Most of the fibre and nutrients are in the skin so cook and eat potatoes unpeeled.

feelings of self-loathing dominate. Various behavioural patterns accompany eating disorders. These include a tendency towards compulsiveness and striving for perfection as well as a fear of sexual development. Although in a few cases there may be a possible genetic or metabolic cause, society's promotion of thinness as attractive is thought to play a very significant role.

Little is known about why certain people suffer eating disorders, although there are some clues provided by its tendency to occur in specific sections of society. Usually, the sufferers are young, female, white and

THE RISKS OF BREAST SURGERY

Unfortunately, it is common for women to be dissatisfied with the size and shape of their breasts, no matter what their figure. Some women feel so strongly that they choose to undergo cosmetic surgery.

Breast enlargement, reduction or mastopexy (breast lift) should not be undertaken lightly or without being properly informed of the risks. All procedures are likely to involve some degree of scarring and also carry the risk of infection, breast pain, loss of sensation and complications for breast-feeding. Implants may move, leak or make the breasts feel unnaturally firm a few years after the operation.

Leakage is a known complication of silicone implants. A link with cancer led to a ban in the US, but recent studies suggest that any risk is so low as to be negligible. Other studies have linked silicone leakage with the development of autoimmune disorders, but these findings are also controversial with many health professionals denying a link.

A more direct danger may be that silicone implants mask the presence of tumours or cysts on mammograms, possibly allowing a developing cancer to go undetected. Women with a strong family history of breast cancer should therefore avoid silicone implants.

A Self-Obsessed Woman

People who become preoccupied with themselves – their body shape, weight and appearance – often have an underlying sense of inadequacy. Controlling their bodies allows them power over their lives. Taken to extreme, this tunnel-visioned effort towards 'perfection' can become obsessive, taking away all pleasure and only serving to fuel insecurities and place excessive pressures on body and mind.

Jilly is an ambitious 35-year-old sales manager. She has a 'driven' personality and works long hours building up her client list. Her staff find her demanding and notice her absence at social gatherings. Jilly goes to the gym every night, where she is just as demanding of herself physically as she is professionally. Jilly is intelligent and attractive, but finds it hard to start a relationship and often gets lonely. She doesn't tell people about her problems because she appears so successful. During a weekend visit to Pam, an old school friend, Jilly confessed how unhappy she was. Pam advised her to stop being so hard on herself and those around her. Jilly found this difficult to accept but promised Pam she would think about it.

WHAT SHOULD JILLY DO?

Jilly needs to accept that she is pushing herself too hard – the expectations she feels she has to live up to are only her own. Her need to control herself and everyone around her is narrowing her life and her demanding physical workouts are a symptom of her driving need for perfection. If she relinquishes some control her life will open up of its own accord. She needs to talk about how she is feeling and decide on some areas that she can change. In order to relax more she should avoid going to the gym so much where she tends to work herself to exhaustion. She should investigate ways of exercising that she might find more enjoyable and start saying 'yes' to social invitations.

Action Plan

WORK
Try to take a more relaxed attitude towards work goals and focus on team-building and cooperation as a means to achieving them.

FITNESS
Cut down on gym visits and workout lengths. Look at more sociable ways of exercising: join a team sport or walking group.

EMOTIONAL HEALTH
Life shouldn't be all work and no play. Make some time to build a social network and relate to people on an emotional level.

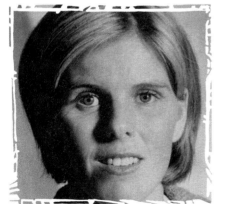

WORK
Making working life enjoyable for others is part of being a good manager. Work is important – but it is only one part of life.

FITNESS
Using exercise as a means of control is dangerous. Never push yourself to reach unachievable goals.

EMOTIONAL HEALTH
Making yourself physically perfect won't automatically lead to fulfilling relationships.

HOW THINGS TURNED OUT FOR JILLY

Jilly began to realise she was obsessive and felt relief once she acknowledged that she didn't have to outperform everyone. Her change in attitude made her more open and people at work began to notice that she was more relaxed and willing to give, rather than demand. She began to focus on her personal relationships, which is paying off in a more enjoyable lifestyle, such as joining a friendly walking group.

STEPS TO IMPROVE SELF-IMAGE

A positive self-image is important for everyone. Insecurities about looks are usually unfounded, but can still leave us feeling miserable and inadequate. Follow these steps towards a happier self:

▶ *Work out your BMI (see page 16) – you may not realise that your weight is healthy.*

▶ *Buy clothes that flatter your shape and disguise problem areas (see Chapter 3).*

▶ *Exercise regularly. Exercise releases 'feel good' endorphins which lift your mood during just one session.*

▶ *Don't put yourself in a situation which makes you feel inadequate. If you are the only one overweight in an aerobics class full of the superfit, change classes.*

middle class. It is estimated that approximately 1 in every 100 people in this group suffers an eating disorder. This figure rises among those who use their bodies professionally – dancers, models, actresses, and female athletes – to a ratio of 1 in 20.

Although there are numerous theories about the psychological aspects of eating disorders, the medical profession – and often the sufferers themselves – cannot truly say why they have such an unhappy relationship with food and their bodies.

Eating disorder sufferers must seek professional help. Left untreated, severe damage can be done to the body; in the worst case, death can occur through starvation. The first line of attack will probably be a course of antidepressants, followed by specialist counselling and/or psychotherapy. The underlying psychological factors will be explored and nutritional supervision will be provided to re-educate the sufferer's eating habits. These treatments may last for several years. Severe cases may require hospitalisation and supervised convalescence.

Recovery from an eating disorder is a long, slow and not always permanent process. Sufferers may find that alternative therapies help to support their medical care. Hypnotherapy may help to identify the causes of the distorted self-image. Autosuggestion aims to nurture a more positive view about body shape and size, and acupuncture can help to relieve stress and rebalance the body's energy.

FEELING GOOD ABOUT YOUR BODY SHAPE

While anorexia and bulimia are still quite rare illnesses, emotional fixations on weight and shape are common. Numerous studies have revealed the extent to which people's sense of self-worth is dangerously linked to their appearance. While feeling good about your appearance does contribute to self-confidence, it's important to keep a preoccupation with shape in perspective. No one is exclusively defined by their appearance; personality, intelligence, outlook and beliefs all combine to make you who you are.

SHAPING UP AND THE 'IDEAL' BODY

It is important to keep your shaping-up goals realistic and not be influenced by the media's portrayal of an 'ideal' shape which may not be healthy for you. Being thin doesn't mean you are healthy – in fact having too small an amount of body fat can put your health at risk. A lot can be achieved through a carefully planned shaping-up programme, but it is vital to keep your perspective of a healthy shape.

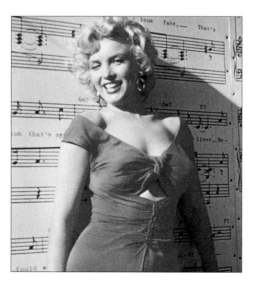

MARILYN MONROE
The womanly curves may not be considered fashionable, but Marilyn's sex appeal is still as strong as ever.

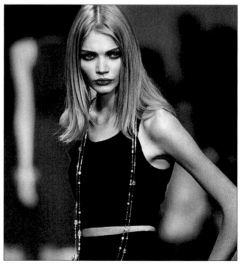

JODIE KIDD
Personifying the 'waif' look of the 1990s fashion world, model Jodie Kidd has been accused of being anorexic.

CHAPTER 2

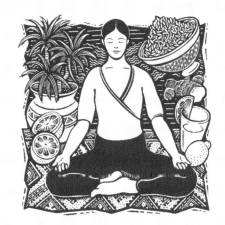

READING YOUR BODY SHAPE

*Your body is, in many ways, a physical record of the
psychological and emotional stresses that you
experience during life. Learning to read your shape
can provide vital information about your attitudes
and major methods of coping. This chapter looks at
a range of body reading therapies, and how they can
reveal and address underlying tensions that hinder
the development of healthy posture and shape.*

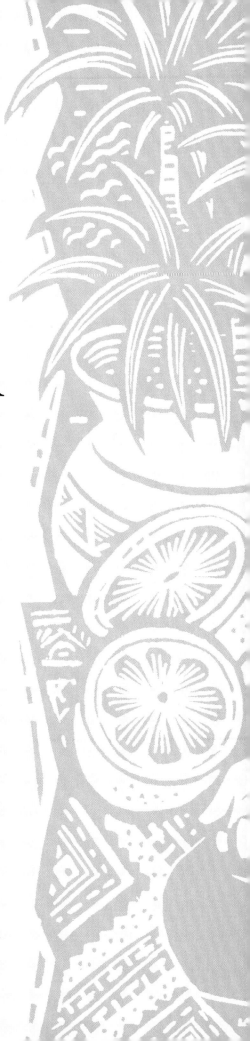

BODY READING

Body reading techniques are used in both Eastern and Western therapies and play an important part in revealing emotional, psychological and physical problems that need to be addressed.

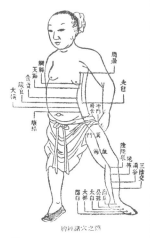

ENERGY MERIDIANS
This Chinese drawing represents one of the main meridian lines used in acupuncture. It is believed that life energy or 'chi' flows along these paths – and its free, unrestricted flow is vital for an aligned and centred body.

CLASS PRESSURE
These pupils are too intent on their exam papers to worry about the well-being of their backs as they write. Schools tend to do little to encourage good posture while students are working. In fact, as here, the space saving is often given priority in classroom design.

At birth, you enter the world programmed with a basic shape derived from the genetic blueprint you inherit from your parents. In a small percentage of cases, genetic or developmental abnormalities leave their mark, but in most cases your physical shape is as unblemished as it is ever going to be. From birth, this basic form will be reshaped by a variety of physical forces that act upon it, such as injury, disease and diet, and occupational factors such as working in a physically demanding job, exercise habits and current fashions. Psychological and emotional factors play an important part in shaping your physical form, too. Tension is a major factor, but other types of inner conflict will also be mirrored in your outward appearance.

The ability to gauge a person's psychological and emotional state of health from a study of physical shape is called body reading and is a vital part in many Eastern therapies, such as Tui Na, t'ai chi and shiatsu. Body reading is also important in many complementary and alternative health therapies that have developed in the West, such as Rolfing, chiropractic, osteopathy, bioenergetics and neo-Reichian therapy.

STRESS AND THE BODY

Your body reflects your emotional state, mental attitude and physical condition through the way that you sit, stand and move around. When you are happy, for example, this is mirrored in freer, bouncier movements and a more erect stance. When you are sad or withdrawn this is shown in a more compressed stance and stiff movements. Physical changes are clearly evident in reaction to stress. Acute stress, such as an injury, accident or tragic news, which shakes your emotional make-up, will immediately affect your posture. Slumped shoulders, a downcast expression and weak knees are common reactions.

Long-term unresolved stress, such as ongoing work or relationship problems, often has a more subtle effect. This is because the postures and facial expressions adopted are designed to mask your inner turmoil so that you can carry on your daily life without drawing attention to your true feelings. Many common expressions reflect this attempt to cope with inner tension: you 'grit your teeth', 'give a fixed smile' and 'carry the weight of the world on your shoulders'.

Constant tension affects various parts of the body in different ways. The face becomes tight and fairly expressionless as the muscles of the mouth, the jaw and eyes stiffen up to hide emotions; the back becomes rigid as the muscles lose flexibility; the head drops forward, putting an uneven load on the neck, which can no longer keep the head balanced so easily; while the shoulders become tense and rounded.

Tension also causes the pelvis to slump forward, putting the spine out of alignment, exaggerating any surplus flesh around the

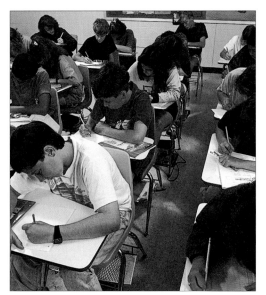

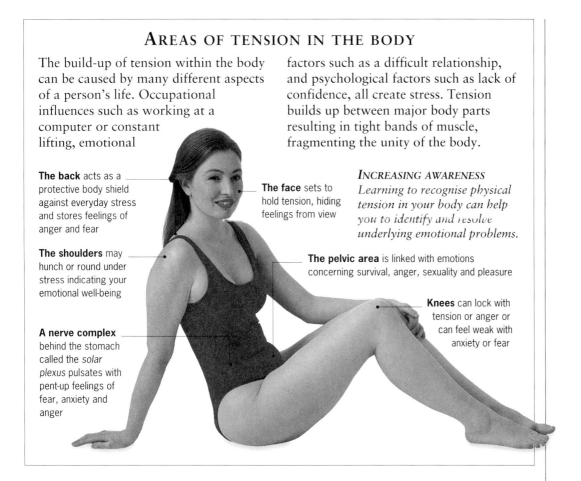

AREAS OF TENSION IN THE BODY

The build-up of tension within the body can be caused by many different aspects of a person's life. Occupational influences such as working at a computer or constant lifting, emotional factors such as a difficult relationship, and psychological factors such as lack of confidence, all create stress. Tension builds up between major body parts resulting in tight bands of muscle, fragmenting the unity of the body.

The back acts as a protective body shield against everyday stress and stores feelings of anger and fear

The shoulders may hunch or round under stress indicating your emotional well-being

A nerve complex behind the stomach called the *solar plexus* pulsates with pent-up feelings of fear, anxiety and anger

The face sets to hold tension, hiding feelings from view

INCREASING AWARENESS
Learning to recognise physical tension in your body can help you to identify and resolve underlying emotional problems.

The pelvic area is linked with emotions concerning survival, anger, sexuality and pleasure

Knees can lock with tension or anger or can feel weak with anxiety or fear

abdominal area. The legs become stiffer and less flexible, which in turn affects balance and creates an unnaturally rigid gait, counteracting the body's natural flowing movements. Chronic tension is a contributory factor to many physical disorders such as back and neckache, facial pain such as myalgia, headaches and migraines, indigestion, stomach ulcers, joint ailments, breathing disorders, and heart problems including cardiac disease.

READING YOUR BODY

Body reading provides a reference system that you can use to evaluate your physical form. Habitual ways of standing reflect your basic persona and can become firmly entrenched. By reading these signs you can judge whether there are deep-seated aspects of your emotional life or psychological profile that you might need to tackle. Subtle abnormalities that might indicate problems are hard to spot in others, but by being more familiar with your own body you can learn to recognise areas that seem, for example, out of alignment, underdeveloped, or abnormally compacted.

In order to read your body from all angles you will need a full-length mirror and a hand-held one, or two large mirrors. Choose a time when you are feeling relaxed. Stand naked in front of the mirror with your back straight and head erect to try to gain an overall impression of your body, and then look at each part of it in turn.

Asymmetries and splits

One important aspect of body reading is the ability to identify asymmetries in the body's overall shape. No one is truly symmetrical. Features on one side of the face will differ marginally from the other, for instance, and your dominant arm is likely to be more developed than the other. A pronounced asymmetry, however, such as an extreme slope to the shoulders or a marked tilt to the hips may indicate a postural fault or a musculoskeletal disorder that may lead to serious physical problems.

If one half of the body seems out of proportion when compared with the other it is called a split. A left/right split occurs when the whole of one side seems noticeably more muscular or better defined than the other,

EYE ASYMMETRY
No one is truly symmetrical and many people have facial asymmetry, particularly in the eyes. On this face, the left eye appears more open, outgoing and receptive while the right eye looks more tense, closed and defensive.

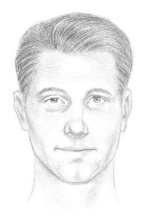

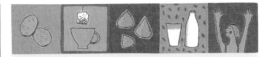

SUPER SHAPER

Made entirely of natural ingredients, fruit and herbal teas present a healthy alternative to tea and coffee. There are a growing variety of flavours available and some have other beneficial properties, for example camomile aids relaxation while lemon invigorates. Although caffeine gives an initial energy boost and can relieve fatigue in the short-term, long-term ingestion, particularly in large amounts (over 5 cups of tea or coffee a day) can actually cause fatigue. In anxiety sufferers, caffeine can increase the levels of anxiety and depression felt, therefore adding to tension held in the body. Tea also has no nutritive value – in fact, it includes tannins which reduce the body's ability to absorb iron.

for example, or softer and more rounded. This may indicate inner conflict between the dominant and passive sides of your nature.

A top/bottom split is closely linked with sexual development. In general, men have broad shoulders and narrow hips and women have the opposite characteristics. A pronounced split is indicated when, allowing for gender differences, the body seems top or bottom-heavy. Top-heavy people tend to be dominating and aggressive while bottom-heavy people are often seen as passive and unassertive.

A front/back split is when the impression created by your front view seems at variance to the back view. For example, your front, which represents the image you wish to show to the world, may seem angular, muscular and well-defined while the back view, representing your hidden feelings, may seem softer, weaker and more vulnerable.

Reading individual body parts

Individual parts of the body also reveal a lot about your emotional profile. Although the face changes expression constantly, certain entrenched characteristics tend to stand out. For example, the eyes may be naturally large and friendly or small and defensive. Sometimes there may be a left/right split, indicating mixed inner feelings. The mouth may be full and relaxed or thin and tense. Tension may be seen in a clenched jaw or furrowed brow. The jaw may thrust forwards, showing aggression or determination, or recede, showing submission.

HOW YOUR PERSONALITY AFFECTS YOUR BODY

Your personality plays a significant part in your shape, posture, stance and movement – in short, your body profile. To understand these influences it is important to make an objective assessment of your personality. Study these body profiles to see whether you recognise any traits of your own. You may identify with more than one.

To make permanent changes to your body profile, you have to change your behaviour. If you recognise any problem areas in your personality, look at the guidelines for change. Change doesn't happen overnight and may be difficult but just accepting your weaknesses is a big step in the right direction.

STOICAL
Seen in people who are under constant stress. As if bearing a heavy burden, their bodies look compressed with a short neck, short torso and stooped shoulders. In addition, the pelvis is tilted forwards and the leg muscles are tight and compacted.

HOW TO CHANGE
You do not have to put up with everything in life. Be prepared to rebel from time to time. When people expect you to put yourself out don't be afraid to say 'no'. State your objections clearly and people will respect you for it.

DEFENSIVE
Common reaction to acute stress or sudden tension such as an argument. The person reacts by contracting inwardly. The shoulders rise and the neck shortens. The arms are held protectively across the body, constricting the chest. The back and legs are held rigid, as if to withstand a sudden onslaught.

HOW TO CHANGE
Don't allow yourself to be browbeaten – make sure your wishes are understood. You need not be aggressive; be patient while the other person makes their case and then state yours. Withdraw if a discussion becomes heated.

The position of the head and neck provides a clear signal of your psychological and emotional state. An erect, forward-angled head may suggest competitiveness, assertiveness and even aggression, especially if accompanied by a jutting jaw. If the head is downcast, however, it may indicate submission or depression. A head held upright appears confident and resolute, while a head held back may be stubborn or defensive. If the head is tilted to one side it can suggest indecision or lack of commitment.

The shoulders and arms may be held back in a way that suggests determination, or pushed forward in a protective posture. Raised shoulders indicate a naturally defensive stance, while drooping shoulders may suggest an acceptance of defeat.

The shape of your chest is determined by your normal breathing pattern and indirectly reflects your psychological profile. An over-inflated chest suggests an outwardly dominant and competitive persona. This might, however, be masking a deep-seated sense of insecurity. A sunken chest may indicate a passive or even defensive person who is unable to let go emotionally.

In Eastern cultures, the abdomen is seen as the seat of the emotions and so is thought to be an important indicator of inner feelings. The abdominal area is also important in body reading for other reasons. The abdominal muscles play a part in all major movements of the upper body and so general tensions or imbalances in the torso will be reflected here, perhaps in a tense and rigid abdomen. The abdominal area is also where excess fat due to overeating is most likely to be deposited, and so may indicate a more general psychological malaise, in which food is an important compensation.

The buttocks and pelvis are associated with sexual feelings. A vertical pelvis with firm but relaxed buttock muscles ensures relaxed and free-flowing movement and reflects a well-balanced temperament. A pelvis that is tilted forwards with loose buttock muscles may indicate weakness and passivity, while a backwards-tilted pelvis and tight buttocks may indicate tension and pent-up emotions.

The legs are important indicators of physical and psychological health. Ideally, the legs should be straight, strong, flexible and evenly balanced to support the body and produce easy, flowing movements. A knock-kneed stance can indicate insecurity, with the legs kept protectively together, making mobility slow and awkward. A bow-legged stance suggests imbalance and uncertainty, making movement more precarious.

continued on page 40

USING BODY LANGUAGE

Your body language can let you down in important situations such as interviews and business meetings. Here are some tips on how to appear open and receptive:

▶ *Holding your head upright with a relaxed jaw suggests confidence. Try to make eye contact as much as you can during the meeting.*

▶ *Don't cross your arms as this can make you appear defensive.*

▶ *Sit tall with your feet firmly on the floor and your shoulders open and relaxed. When engaged in conversation, leaning forwards towards the other person conveys interest.*

▶ *Don't fidget or you will appear nervous.*

▶ *Remember to smile.*

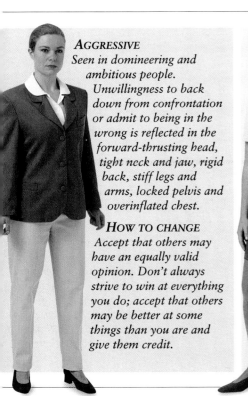

AGGRESSIVE
Seen in domineering and ambitious people. Unwillingness to back down from confrontation or admit to being in the wrong is reflected in the forward-thrusting head, tight neck and jaw, rigid back, stiff legs and arms, locked pelvis and overinflated chest.

HOW TO CHANGE
Accept that others may have an equally valid opinion. Don't always strive to win at everything you do; accept that others may be better at some things than you are and give them credit.

BOASTFUL
These people portray a false confidence and superiority. The head is held too high straining the neck, the chest is puffed out and the stomach constricted. The legs are loose, throwing the back out of alignment.

HOW TO CHANGE
Accept that creating a false impression of your abilities is not fooling anyone – least of all yourself. Play to your strengths but admit to your weaknesses too – you don't have to be perfect.

WITHDRAWN
This profile is shown by people who find it difficult to reveal their emotions. They tense all their muscles and joints creating a protective shield from the outside world. As a result the whole body appears contracted, physically matching the psychological withdrawal.

HOW TO CHANGE
You will not turn into an extrovert overnight, but you will benefit from a more open personality. Be interested in what others are doing. If you make the first move in starting a friendly conversation, you will find it is quickly reciprocated.

The Tui Na Practitioner

Tui Na is a vigorous physical therapy that is used to relieve the build-up of tension in your body, and to treat illness and injury. It can also reveal and help to release emotional factors that may lie behind physical symptoms.

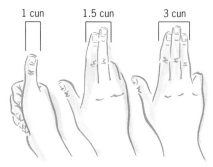

1 cun   1.5 cun   3 cun

MEASURING CHI-POINTS
The cun is a unit used in Chinese medicine to measure the distance of chi-points from the bones and muscles of the body.

Literally meaning 'push and grasp', Tui Na is a massage therapy that has been practised in China for more than 4000 years. Today it is an integral part of the medicinal practices of modern China. Tui Na is a very physical therapy involving deep invigorating massage to release blocked 'life energy', or 'chi'. In Chinese medical theory this energy flows through energy channels, known as meridians, in the body. Tui Na exerts pressure along these meridians and at specific points – known as chi-points – to release any

blockages and enable the chi to flow through the body unhindered. The free distribution of this energy is thought to have enormous effects on a person's well-being, not only physically but emotionally, intellectually and spiritually as well. A Tui Na massage session not only releases the energy of the patient, but also that of the therapist. This mutual releasing and exchanging of chi is thought to be beneficial to both participants.

How do I find a Tui Na therapist?
Tui Na is still emerging as a therapy in the West and so there are not a great number of fully trained therapists working at present. Your local health centre or alternative medicine centre may be able to advise you of any local practitioners. Because Tui Na involves a vigorous massage it is essential to ensure that your therapist is fully qualified.

Who can benefit from Tui Na?
In China, Tui Na massage is used as a therapy on everyone from the age of five upwards. The therapy consists of deep massage, but is used to varying degrees on different people. For example, the same depth of massage would not be used on an elderly person as on a younger person. Infants under five are not regarded as having fully developed meridian systems, so the therapy concentrates on the feet and hands in very young children. Tui Na should not be used by anyone with serious

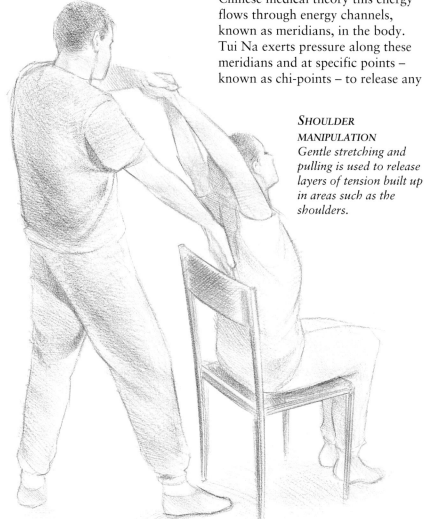

SHOULDER MANIPULATION
Gentle stretching and pulling is used to release layers of tension built up in areas such as the shoulders.

heart disease, cancer (especially of the skin or lymphatic system) or osteoporosis. Tui Na can be adapted during pregnancy – specific points, such as the lower abdomen, should be avoided, however.

Is it a safe therapy?

Tui Na is considered extremely safe, although there may be some bruising in susceptible people. If the wrong point on a meridian is stimulated, no benefit will be gained by the patient, but no harm will be done either; the chi will soon rebalance itself if it is stimulated wrongly.

What sort of problems is Tui Na used to treat?

Traditional Chinese medicine, of which Tui Na is a part, is primarily concerned with preventive medicine, but chronic conditions are treated as well. Chinese medical philosophy sees the progress from health to illness as a journey, along which symptoms can be observed, such as dizziness or nausea. Tui Na or acupuncture can be used to maintain health, and to check more serious ailments before they have a chance to take hold. Tui Na is especially good for treating muscular aches and pains, sports injuries and other symptoms of physical stress on the body. It can also be used to relieve the symptoms of some ailments such as asthma, migraine and irritable bowel syndrome.

How will a consultation start?

Tui Na massage is a holistic therapy that works to benefit your entire body and mind. The therapist will begin by asking you questions about your current state of health and mind, and your lifestyle. From this, he or she will draw conclusions about which meridian lines need to be worked on during the therapy, and more specifically at which points on the meridians the energy may be blocked. It is essential to feel relaxed with the practitioner – communication is important throughout the massage session.

What is involved during a Tui Na massage?

A Tui Na session will usually last for about an hour. The massage will take place fully clothed and does not make use of oils, so you should wear loose, comfortable clothing. A whole body massage will begin with a seated neck and shoulder massage. The practitioner will then ask you to move to a massage table (one without a mattress as this would absorb the beneficial pressure). Sometimes heavy pressure is used which may feel uncomfortable at first, especially if the muscle is particularly tense. The practitioner will usually start with gentler pressure and progress to a deeper and more vigorous massage as your body relaxes. Tui Na should never

cause intense pain, however, and if anything does cause you pain you should tell the therapist immediately.

How will I feel after the treatment?

On the whole, most people feel revitalised and energetic after a Tui Na treatment. However, as Tui Na releases any blocked emotional energy when the flow of chi is stimulated, you may be surprised to find yourself close to tears, or feeling excessively emotional after a treatment. This could even occur up to a couple of days later. If this happens, the Chinese approach to dealing with such emotion is to acknowledge its presence and then release it. This release of feelings is good for your emotional health and well-being.

WHAT YOU CAN DO AT HOME

It is easy to incorporate a Tui Na self-massage into your daily routine. Find a place to relax and make sure your clothing is loose and comfortable. The room should be warm and softly lit as bright lights may prevent your eyes from relaxing.

Start by using your right hand, clenched in a loose fist, to pummel the outside of your left arm up to the shoulder and then down the inside. Repeat this several times and then swap to the other arm. Next, support your right elbow with your left hand and reach over your shoulder to pummel your upper back. Reach back as far as you can. Repeat with the left arm supported by your right hand. Continue this for about a minute, or longer if you prefer. Your back should feel relaxed and tingling.

Next, using both hands, pummel the front of your chest, especially your rib cage, continuing for at least a minute. Next, bend forwards from a standing position and pummel down both sides of your back and buttocks, and then using the heels of your hands vigorously rub the centre of your lower back, in the area where your kidneys are. Remain in

this forward-leaning position and move your legs apart, pummel down the outside and then the inside of both legs simultaneously.

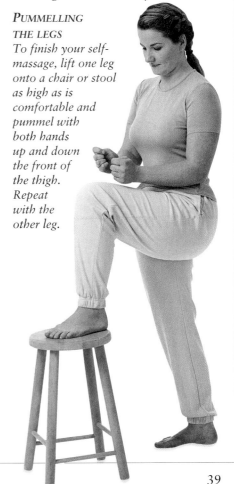

PUMMELLING THE LEGS
To finish your self-massage, lift one leg onto a chair or stool as high as is comfortable and pummel with both hands up and down the front of the thigh. Repeat with the other leg.

The feet are very important in Eastern body reading because they provide contact with the earth and allow energy to flow through the body. This contact is called grounding. In grounded people, the foot is supple and keeps the body balanced by ensuring the weight is evenly distributed. In ungrounded people, the foot is weak and flat, or rigid and excessively arched, leaving them unbalanced, unsteady and slow to react.

PRACTICAL STEPS TO CHANGING YOUR BODY PROFILE

Once you have learnt how to recognise the negative influences on your body profile, you will more than likely have found areas that you want to change – perhaps in your day-to-day behaviour, the way you react to particular situations, how you move, or the way you hold yourself throughout the day. There are many practical things you can do to bring about change, but bear in mind that this will require patience: transitions in the way we move or think are a re-education process and do not happen overnight.

However, simply being aware of your posture, paying attention to it and thinking about how you use your body is a big step in the direction of change. You will be able to recognise personality traits and the areas of your body where tension is being held. By giving some thought to why this tension is present, you may be able to resolve deep-seated problems and find your way to a happier self.

Learning to relax

Being able to relax is essential in order to reduce stress levels and can go a long way to avoiding build-up of stress and negative character traits, making you more able to cope with the challenges of daily life. In the first instance, learn to control your breathing. Sit or lie down in a warm, comfortable room and breathe slowly and deeply from the abdomen. Feel your chest expand to its maximum capacity and then hold the breath briefly before slowly releasing it again. Keep breathing deeply until you feel the tension drain from your body.

CORRECTING YOUR SITTING POSTURE

Many people spend a large proportion of their lives in a seated position. Sitting puts one-third more pressure on the spine than standing and poor seated posture, often encouraged by badly designed chairs, can result in a build-up of tension in the body and lead to back complaints. A prolonged seated position leads to muscle fatigue causing you to slump down farther into your chair as the day progresses. Use the guide below to check and correct your sitting position and keep reminding yourself throughout the day. To reduce muscle fatigue, allow time regularly during the day to stand up and walk around or do a few stretches.

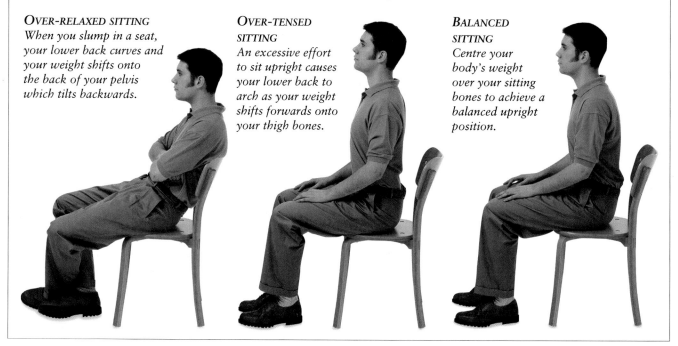

OVER-RELAXED SITTING
When you slump in a seat, your lower back curves and your weight shifts onto the back of your pelvis which tilts backwards.

OVER-TENSED SITTING
An excessive effort to sit upright causes your lower back to arch as your weight shifts forwards onto your thigh bones.

BALANCED SITTING
Centre your body's weight over your sitting bones to achieve a balanced upright position.

RELAXING THROUGH VISUALISATION

This visualisation exercise can form part of a tension-releasing regime. Allow about 15 minutes for the exercise. Picture a scene that you find calming, perhaps a sunny, secluded beach, or a tranquil lake. Imagine yourself as an object within that scene; perhaps a piece of driftwood moving lazily with the tide. You are responsive to movement but remain unchanged.

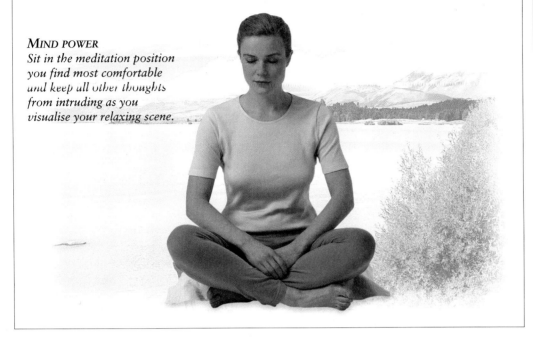

MIND POWER
Sit in the meditation position you find most comfortable and keep all other thoughts from intruding as you visualise your relaxing scene.

The next step is to ease the tension in your muscles. Focus on the muscles of each part of the body in turn, tightening them as you inhale and then slowly relaxing them as you exhale. Start with the muscles in your feet and work up your body, bit by bit, to finish with the face muscles. By the end of this session all the muscles in your body will feel much more relaxed. Try to set aside at least 30 minutes each day for a period of total relaxation or meditation.

Changing your posture
Once you feel mentally and physically more relaxed you should concentrate on making improvements in your posture. To keep your body in perfect alignment it needs to be balanced. Keep your back and neck straight and your head erect as you sit, stand or walk, so that your upper body weight is carried directly over your spine. When seated, rest your hands in your lap or on the arms of the chair, and let them hang easily at your sides as you stand and walk. Keep your movements fluid and your knees, hips and elbows loose. Roll your feet from your heels to your toes as you walk, always remembering to keep your head up, your eyes looking straight ahead and your body evenly balanced over your legs.

Regular exercise
Long-term stress can lead to entrenched changes in physical shape and posture that will require a programme of targeted exercises to sort out. Regular physical exercise such as brisk walking, jogging, dancing, or an active sport, will keep your musculoskeletal system loose and relaxed and improve the circulation to the tissues and joints, providing vital nutrients and allowing wastes to flow away easily. Start the day with a short period of limbering up exercise such as jogging on the spot or a series of easy stretches. This will loosen the joints and increase the blood flow to the head, helping to clear your mind of tension in preparation for the day ahead.

At the end of a stressful day, dance to your favourite up-tempo music or shake out the tension in your body (see right). Follow this with a warm, relaxing bath, perhaps adding a few drops each of lavender and rosemary aromatherapy oils.

RELEASING TENSION
Shaking out your muscles is an ideal way to release tension at the end of a stressful day. It can also be used as a wake-up call for your muscles first thing in the morning, as part of a warm-up before exercise, or to shake out muscles after exercise.

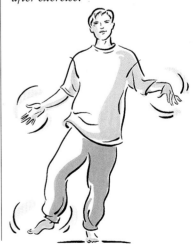

AYURVEDA AND BODY SHAPES

Body reading is an integral part of Ayurveda, an ancient health system originating in India, which diagnoses health complaints in the context of body type.

Ayurveda is one of the oldest medical systems in the world and has been practised in India for over 4000 years. It is believed to be based on the accumulated knowledge of holy men called *rishis*, or seers of truth, who gained religious and philosophical enlightenment through religious practices and disciplines. This knowledge of life is described in the scriptures of the Vedas, the most ancient of the Hindu holy texts. Many of the established Eastern systems of philosophy and medicine have been heavily influenced by the principles of Ayurvedic medicine. This is why it is sometimes referred to as 'the mother of all healing'.

Ayurvedic medicine takes a holistic – whole body – approach to health, recognising that many physical symptoms can reflect more wide-ranging and apparently unconnected problems, such as physical misalignments, internal blockages, psychological ailments, and dietary or digestive disorders. Ayurvedic practitioners do not treat symptoms directly but use a combination of therapies including herbal medicines, massage, diet and yoga to correct the imbalances that are causing the underlying disorders.

THE THREE BODY TYPES: VATA, PITTA AND KAPHA

In Ayurvedic theory, all people are governed by three natural forces, or doshas: vata, the force of air and movement; pitta, the force of fire and energy; and kapha, the force of earth and growth. It is the combination, balance or imbalance of these three forces in all individuals that accounts for their metabolism, their body shape and their likelihood of developing any kind of physical disorder.

Typical vata body types are thin, with prominent features and cool, dry skin. They are imaginative and highly active people who show flashes of intuition but can be moody. They are prone to nervous disorders, such as stress and anxiety attacks, depression, high blood pressure, sleeplessness, stomach upsets and cramps.

Pitta types are fair with a medium build and a ruddy complexion. They tend to be organised, efficient and warm-hearted but can also be short-tempered and intense. Pitta people are prone to skin conditions such as eczema, sleep disorders, aggressive behaviour, piles, gallstones, stomach ulcers and heartburn.

continued on page 44

HEALTH THROUGH KNOWLEDGE

Ayurvedic practitioners believe that only when body, mind and soul are in harmony is complete health possible. The health system takes account of the human's relationship with the heavens and the cosmos and encompasses science, religion and philosophy. The name Ayurveda literally means 'science of life' from *Ayu* meaning life and *veda* meaning knowledge. In order for us to receive this knowledge, traditionally reserved for the Gods and the enlightened, the three doshas – vata, pitta and kapha – must be in balance, a state achieved through practising Ayurveda.

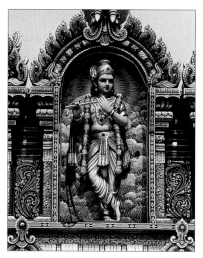

KNOWLEDGE OF THE GODS
Ayurvedic philosophy states that all knowledge comes from the almighty Hindu god, Krishna.

HOW TO DETERMINE YOUR AYURVEDIC BODY TYPE

The following questionnaire can help you to determine which Ayurvedic body type, or types, matches you most closely. Starting with vata, look at each of the characteristics listed and circle the figure that you feel is most appropriate to you. Add up the results of the test so that you have a total figure. Do the pitta and kapha tests in the same way until you have a total for each of the three sections then look at 'how to score'.

VATA

	RARELY	SOMETIMES	OFTEN
Light build	0	1	2
Quick to act	0	1	2
Poor memory	0	1	2
Slow to decide	0	1	2
Quick to learn	0	1	2
Lively	0	1	2
Enthusiastic	0	1	2
Excitable	0	1	2
Energetic	0	1	2
Receptive to ideas	0	1	2
Talkative	0	1	2
Sensitive to cold	0	1	2
Anxious	0	1	2
Irregular eating and sleeping habits	0	1	2
Changing moods	0	1	2
Total			

PITTA

	RARELY	SOMETIMES	OFTEN
Medium build	0	1	2
Hearty eater	0	1	2
Efficient	0	1	2
Punctilious	0	1	2
Regular habits	0	1	2
Strong willed	0	1	2
Irritable	0	1	2
Intolerant	0	1	2
Impatient	0	1	2
Blunt speaking	0	1	2
Tenacious	0	1	2
Self-critical	0	1	2
Enjoy a challenge	0	1	2
Dislike warm, humid weather	0	1	2
Sweat easily	0	1	2
Total			

KAPHA

	RARELY	SOMETIMES	OFTEN
Heavy build	0	1	2
Prone to overweight	0	1	2
Abundant, thick dark hair	0	1	2
Smooth, pale skin	0	1	2
Calm and placid	0	1	2
Sound sleeper	0	1	2
Slow to anger	0	1	2
Slow to learn	0	1	2
Good memory	0	1	2
Good with money	0	1	2
Dislike being cold	0	1	2
Gentle	0	1	2
Cheerful	0	1	2
Affectionate	0	1	2
Slow eater	0	1	2
Total			

HOW TO SCORE

To find your dominating dosha, compare your scores for the three tests and decide if one outweighs the other two, or if two dosha types predominate. Perhaps all three scores are quite close together? Use the following example results as a guide:

Vata 20, Pitta 18, Kapha 10 = Vata-pitta type

Vata 23, Pitta 10, Kapha 5 = Vata type

Vata 9, Pitta 8, Kapha 7 = Vata-pitta-kapha type

Vata 10, Pitta 8, Kapha 22 = Kapha type

Vata 10, Pitta 17, Kapha 19 = Pitta-kapha type

When you have worked out your dosha type, you will be able to apply Ayurveda more accurately to your lifestyle. However, to understand the full significance of your body type, it is best to seek the advice of an experienced Ayurvedic practitioner, especially if your characteristics are spread across the three types more or less equally.

TEN-DAY PURIFICATION DIET

The first step in practising Ayurveda is a ten-day purification diet of light, easily digested foods. A practitioner will devise a diet tailored to your dosha or the diet shown here can be used as part of a self-help programme. The diet will improve digestion and allow your body to expel the toxins and waste products known as *ama* in Ayurvedic terms. Listed below are the foods allowed during the diet and brief diet guidelines. After ten days, gradually start to eat normally, following a diet suitable to your dosha type.

▶ *Fruits: oranges, bananas, mango and papaya. Oranges should be sucked rather than eaten in segments as this aids salivation and boosts the metabolism.*

▶ *Vegetables: potatoes, carrots, broccoli, beetroot, cooked leaf vegetables, cauliflower.*

▶ *Pulses: lentils, rice, wheat and mung beans, the last being particularly high in protein.*

▶ *Flavourings: turmeric and ginger.*

▶ *The only bread allowed is chapatti made with wholemeal flour.*

▶ *Avoid roast, fried, fatty, sour and uncooked foods; fish, pork and beef; cheese, yoghurt and other milk products and sweet food.*

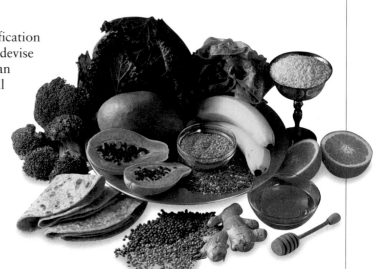

DIET GUIDELINES

On waking and at intervals during the day, drink warm, boiled water with a little lemon and honey added. This stimulates the metabolism and the elimination of *ama*. During the diet it is recommended that you miss breakfast unless you are very hungry when you could eat a chapatti or drink some freshly squeezed fruit juice. Lunch should be the main meal of the day and consist of a light, warm meal such as rice and vegetables. Miss dinner or have a light meal – fruit juice or a small bowl of soup made with grains or vegetables.

Those who fit the kapha type are heavily built with thick, wavy hair and pale skin. They are easy-going, compassionate and affectionate but lack motivation and are prone to allergies, obesity and heart disease.

Each dosha has a seat in a particular part of the body. Vata is based in the large intestine, bones, ears and thighs; pitta is found in the small intestine, stomach and blood; and kapha is found in the chest, lungs and spinal fluid. All three doshas exist in the body in combinations that match the individual's constitution. According to Ayurvedic medicine, when these doshas are balanced in accordance with the individual's personality, that person is fit and healthy, but when the doshas are out of balance, physical and mental disorders arise. Ayurvedic medicine aims to restore the doshas to equilibrium.

AYURVEDIC THERAPY

An Ayurvedic practitioner will recommend a daily health regime tailored to your body type and physical condition or disorder.

The practitioner may recommend starting with a ten-day purification diet designed to rid the body of waste products and harmful toxins, known as *ama*. This might comprise one or two light meals each day consisting of rice, cooked vegetables, beans and soup, but avoiding meat and fish, dairy products and fried or roasted foods.

Foods for dosha types

After this ten-day period, the regular diet will be based on the individual's constitution type in order to balance the dominating dosha. For example, vata types should have stews, pasta, rice, wheat and baked dishes but avoid salads, raw vegetables and most pulses. Vata types are prone to digestive problems so it is important that meals are easily digestible. People of this type should also ensure that they eat in a pleasant environment as they are sensitive to stress. Pitta types should eat vegetables, fruit, dairy products, poultry and game but avoid all red meat, yoghurt and hot spices. Pitta types can overeat and may take the edge off their appetite with bitter and astringent foods or eating regularly and not skipping meals. Kapha types should eat low-fat spicy dishes, fresh fruit, vegetables, and pulses but avoid rice, wheat and most meats. Cold weather can unbalance kapha types, so in winter hot and spicy foods are recommended.

Whole body massage

Another aspect of Ayurveda is regular massage with oils to stimulate the elimination of toxins and waste products by increasing the blood circulation. Massage is also therapeutic, relaxing the body and mind. Massage should be a regular part of your morning routine – vata types should include a daily period of self-massage whereas for pitta and kapha types two or three times a week is sufficient. High-quality cold-pressed sesame oil is recommended, but pitta types and those with skin complaints are recommended to use olive, coconut or sweet almond oil instead. You can find these oils in pharmacists and health food shops.

To improve the oil's suitability for massage and lengthen its storage life, heat it gently for a few minutes in a saucepan to

Pathway to health

Yogic exercises or *asanas* are an important part of Ayurvedic practice, helping to unite the body and mind and balance the three doshas. The *asanas* aim to ease tensed muscles, tone the internal organs and improve flexibility. If you are completely new to yoga, you will find it very helpful to attend a class – many adult education and sports centres run classes for all levels of ability ranging from beginners to advanced. The teacher will be able to assess your capabilities and advise you on correct execution. As the weeks go by, your flexibility will improve immensely and you will gain enough knowledge to practise the exercises safely at home as part of a daily routine.

about 110°C (230°F). Use a thermometer to check the temperature or add a couple of drops of water to the hot oil – if it sizzles the temperature is about right. Prepare about 150 ml (5 fl oz) of oil at a time and decant it

SPORTS FOR DOSHA TYPES

Ayurvedic exercise aims for balance between body and mind and tends to be gentle and enriching, without placing undue stress on the body. Walks in the countryside and controlled exercises such as yoga are ideal. Ayurvedic exercise can take the form of sport but would not be competitive. Furthermore, not all sports are thought to be suitable for all dosha types – your physique and personality type make you more suited to certain activities than others.

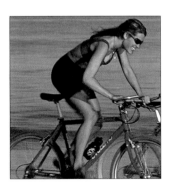

ENERGETIC VATA
Slim and energetic, vata types are best at aerobics, cycling, walking and rambling, and more graceful forms of dancing such as ballet.

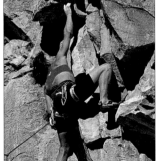

QUICK-WITTED PITTA
Medium-built pitta types are suited to jogging, horse riding, orienteering, swimming, mountaineering and skiing.

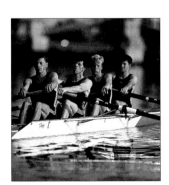

PERSEVERING KAPHA
These are suited to sports requiring control and endurance such as fencing, football, running, rowing, tennis and weightlifting.

ALTERNATE NOSTRIL BREATHING

To achieve rhythmic breathing, Ayurveda recommends the yogic practice of alternate nostril breathing or *pranayama*. Wear loose, comfortable clothing and sit easily in a cross-legged position or in a chair with your back and neck straight but not tense. Close your eyes and breathe deeply a few times, concentrating on the breath in your nostrils. When you are ready, open your eyes and follow steps 1 and 2 below. Continue the sequence for about 5 minutes, then finish by sitting still for a minute breathing normally.

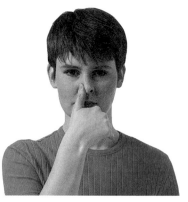

1 *Lightly close the airway of your right nostril with your right thumb. Breathe out slowly through your open left nostril. Breathe in after a few seconds through the left nostril then pinch the nostril shut.*

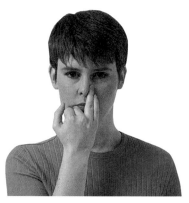

2 *At the same time, release the right nostril and the air you are holding. Breathe out slowly through the right nostril and hold your breath for a few seconds. Breathe in, close the nostril shut again and repeat the process.*

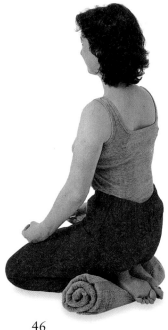

EASY MEDITATION POSE
This yoga pose is an ideal position for breathing and meditation exercises. Kneel with your feet straight and your sitting bones resting evenly on your heels. Placing a rolled blanket under your feet and/or a cushion over your heels may improve comfort and enable you to maintain the position for longer.

into an airtight jar for future use. Apply the oil all over the body so that it can be absorbed by the skin before the massage begins. The body is then massaged from head to foot using gentle, circular movements of the hands.

Yogic exercise

Regular yoga exercises (see page 138) are an important element of Ayurvedic therapy. Yoga enhances suppleness and mobility, eases muscle tension, and can alleviate disorders such as headaches and migraines, back pain, stiff joints and circulatory disorders. A yoga session will usually begin with stretches and bending movements to prepare the body, followed by the adoption of special body positions, or *asanas*. Regular, even and deep breathing is an important part of yoga sessions.

Breathing and meditation

Ayurveda stresses the importance of proper breathing. The alternate nostril breathing exercise (above), called *pranayama*, is designed to control and enhance the natural energy flow, or *prana,* in the body, leading to good health. Practised for 5 minutes each morning and evening the exercise prepares the body for the final stage of the Ayurvedic regime – meditation.

Just as *ama,* or physical waste products, can build up in the body, so too can emotional wastes. Meditation is the process by which the body rids itself of this emotional *ama.* A daily meditation session of 15 minutes is usually sufficient, although it can be longer. Choose a comfortable position – those practised at yoga such as the lotus position – or sit upright in a chair with your back straight. Rest your hands on your thighs or in your lap. It may help to have an object near such as a candle to focus on at first. Breathe calmly as you look at the candle and then close your eyes and hold the image in your head, letting your thoughts drift. Don't try to control your thoughts or stop other thoughts intruding, but don't dwell on anything. As your thoughts become more unfocused, breathe more deeply. To end the session, rest quietly for a few moments with your eyes open while you evaluate any changes you have experienced in yourself.

BODY READING THERAPIES

Body reading therapies aim to identify and relieve the underlying mental and emotional problems which can be causing physical disorders, bad posture and restricted movement.

Most therapies take account of the physical symptoms of a disorder in order to arrive at a diagnosis. But some forms of therapy, sometimes known as body reading therapies, also put great store on close study of the patient's posture in order to discover any underlying cause of the physical condition.

Body reading therapies are based on the belief that there is a close connection between a patient's emotional and psychological problems and that person's stance and movement patterns. By correcting any faults in the patient's posture and way of moving – the physical manifestations of the problem – the therapist aims to alleviate the underlying problem itself. The Alexander technique and Rolfing are two of the most widely practised body reading therapies. Other similar techniques, such as Hellerwork, Looyenwork and Watsu, are also gaining in popularity.

ALEXANDER TECHNIQUE

One of the first people to recognise the connection between inner psychological states and outward physical problems was not a therapist at all but an actor, called Frederick Matthias Alexander. Alexander began to lose his voice when on stage and yet not

---

ALEXANDER TECHNIQUE APPLIED TO SWIMMING

The Alexander technique can highlight ways to improve posture and movement during activities to avoid build-up of pressure and tension. The most common fault in swimming is to swim with your head out of water which puts pressure on the spine. Practice or tuition can help you to overcome this problem and to establish a breathing pattern, which will also improve your swimming technique.

▶ *Invest in some good-quality goggles to protect your eyes from the chlorine in the water. Practise with them in shallow water so that you can stand at any time.*

▶ *To avoid gasping when you lift your head out of the water to inhale, practise exhaling while your head is under the water; releasing the air from your mouth very slowly.*

▶ *Gradually increase the number of strokes you do with your head under water. In front crawl, your goal is to do four or five strokes, then lift your head to the side for a breath.*

▶ *By swimming with your head level with your body, you maintain correct body alignment and achieve better forward propulsion.*

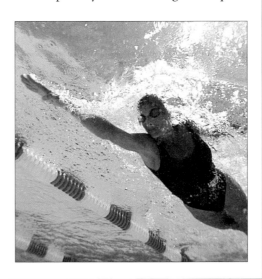

---

at other times, and so he studied himself while rehearsing in front of a mirror to see if he could discover the cause of the problem. He noticed that the stress of acting caused him to shrink down into himself, lowering his head, which constricted his neck and throat and obstructed his breathing. By constantly observing himself and consciously correcting the postural faults he detected, he was able to reduce his feelings of stress, restore his normal voice and develop a healthier, more natural posture.

Alexander developed his observations into a comprehensive therapy – the Alexander technique, which became very popular, particularly among actors and orators, and is now widely practised in Europe and America. The technique aims to improve posture and mobility and promote physical and mental harmony. It is most often used to relieve anxiety and stress and to alleviate back and neck pain, but can also be used to treat headaches, high blood pressure, respiratory conditions, intestinal disorders such as irritable bowel syndrome, and arthritis.

Before starting treatment, an Alexander technique teacher will study the way the patient sits, stands and walks. They will be looking for postural errors such as a slouching or round-shouldered stance, arched or stiff back, or a head held too far back.

While the patient is seated or standing, the teacher then very gently manipulates the body into the correct alignment and gives advice on healthy posture. The teacher also explains how to recognise and relieve stress. For lasting physical benefits it is important that the subject puts the teacher's advice into practice during daily life, and not just in the treatment room.

ROLFING

Rolfing uses massage and manipulation techniques to improve posture and alleviate deep-seated tension, chronic muscle and joint problems and other physical ailments.

Rolfing is sometimes called deep-tissue bodywork, because the therapist manipulates the deep muscular and connective tissues as well as the surface tissues of the body. In particular, Rolfing concentrates on a form of connective tissue called fascia which surrounds the muscles and muscle fibres and also thickens to form tendons.

American biochemist Dr Ida Rolf, the founder of Rolfing, discovered that fascia tissue adapts to your posture and movement patterns, and can become fixed, locking you into bad postural habits. For example, if you habitually hunch your shoulders the fascia will tighten into this position, making it difficult to break the habit.

Dr Rolf believed that to improve your shape, the fascia would have to be stretched and manipulated into the correct positions using various Rolfing techniques so that the connective tissue adapts to the change and supports you in the new healthy posture.

Many postural problems that cause the body to be out of alignment are believed to be caused by deep-seated emotional traumas. For example, feeling depressed could cause you to adopt a round-shouldered and compacted shape. Dr Rolf believed that by correcting these postural problems she could also release the emotional traumas that caused them in the first place.

A skilled Rolfer will study the way the patient sits, stands and walks around to diagnose misalignments that will need to be corrected. A photograph is taken of

AREAS OF
MISALIGNMENT
Body reading therapies including Rolfing, the Alexander technique and osteopathy will start with a complete posture assessment. The practitioner will look at the alignment of your body while you are standing, sitting and walking. This picture shows some common areas of misalignment. Here, the person's weight is shifted onto the left side putting stress on the weightbearing joints of the knee and ankle. In an effort to compensate, the spine becomes curved and the ribs on the left side are cramped, restricting breathing.

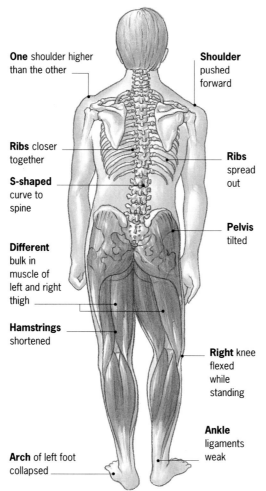

One shoulder higher than the other

Ribs closer together

S-shaped curve to spine

Different bulk in muscle of left and right thigh

Hamstrings shortened

Arch of left foot collapsed

Shoulder pushed forward

Ribs spread out

Pelvis tilted

Right knee flexed while standing

Ankle ligaments weak

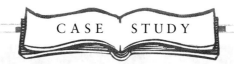
The Unassertive Secretary

Unassertive people often get taken for granted. They may be given tasks that others complain about and even passed over for promotion in favour of less able but more assertive people. This leads to frustration that manifests itself in physical ailments such as chronic muscle pain and headaches. Treating the symptoms alone is not sufficient – a fundamental change in attitude is required.

Jan is a 45-year-old secretary at a pharmaceutical company and has worked for her current boss for over 11 years. Jan is regarded as a conscientious worker by colleagues: she is prepared to put in long hours without complaint, and often takes on extra unpaid tasks, such as organising company social events. Despite her good reputation within the company she has never been offered promotion to a more senior level and has seen other, less experienced people promoted above her. Her lack of progress has left her increasingly despondent and she has started suffering from regular headaches and pain in her shoulder. Recently the pain has prevented her from playing in her regular weekly tennis match.

WHAT SHOULD JAN DO?

Jan's aches and pains are most likely stress-related and linked to feelings of low self-esteem. Because of her lack of assertiveness, others at work take her for granted. Unless she can alter her basic personality profile this situation is unlikely to change. Jan needs to assert herself more, and also needs to redress the balance of work and relaxation in her life, taking more time for her own interests, as well as her health needs. Reintroducing regular exercise into her life might help her to manage her pain better. A friend suggested that Hellerwork might help as the therapy looks at underlying emotional and psychological problems as well as physical disorders.

Action Plan

WORK
Attend course to learn how to confront colleagues and managers positively about areas of dissatisfaction.

EMOTIONAL HEALTH
Accept that unexpressed emotions need to be released somehow. Learn how to use assertion to express feelings in a positive way.

FITNESS
Allocate time each day to some form of exercise, such as yoga, aimed at relieving tension and stretching muscles.

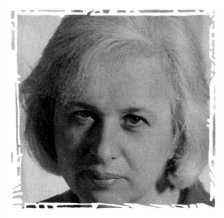

FITNESS
Neglecting to exercise regularly can exacerbate muscle tension.

WORK
Being unassertive at work can lead to missed promotions and a lack of recognition, in the long term causing frustration and anger.

EMOTIONAL HEALTH
Repressed emotions can cause tension in the body which can lead to misalignments of posture and painful muscle problems.

HOW THINGS TURNED OUT FOR JAN

The Hellerworker's analysis revealed long-held anger and frustration. He used massage and manipulation to ease the muscle tension and talked to Jan about the need to release her pent-up feelings. He also prescribed daily exercises. After the first session Jan felt quite emotional, and thought hard about areas of dissatisfaction in her life. By the end of the course her pain had improved and she resolved to take an assertiveness course.

Origins

Hellerwork was the brainchild of former aerospace engineer, Joseph Heller. It is closely based on Rolfing, the bodywork system founded in the mid 1960s by the American biochemist Dr Ida Rolf (1896–1979). Heller studied under Dr Rolf and was the first president of the Rolf Institute in 1976 before leaving to set up his own system of bodywork therapy. This combines tissue manipulation with posture and movement education, and also places emphasis on understanding the memories and attitudes that are released during sessions.

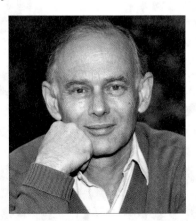

JOSEPH HELLER
Hellerwork therapists explore any memories and emotions released during the sessions by questioning the client about their feelings throughout the therapy.

LOOYENWORK

The theory that psychological trauma is stored in the physical body is explored to a greater degree in Looyenwork. This body reading therapy was founded by Ted Looyen, a psychotherapist, who failed to find relief for his own chronic back pain in massage and manipulation therapies.

Looyenwork uses physical manipulation, but it is directed more at relieving chronic emotional tension and resolving psychological conflicts, such as those arising from divorce or parental rejection. The therapist reads the way the subject sits and stands, and how his or her muscles move to uncover these deep-seated traumas. Patients are counselled on the emotional changes that they are undergoing while the therapist manipulates the body to alleviate the outward physical signs of emotional tension. In addition, therapists aim to enhance the patients' confidence, self-esteem and concentration.

the patient before treatment begins to highlight the problem areas, such as stooped shoulders or arched back. Another picture is taken after the course of treatment has been completed to show the changes that Rolfing has brought about.

As well as improved posture and relief from physical problems such as neck and back pain, patients who have undergone a course of treatment often report increased energy and vitality.

HELLERWORK

Hellerwork is a form of deep-tissue body work with many similarities to Rolfing. It was originated by Joseph Heller who trained with Dr Rolf before devising his own therapy system.

The main difference between the two forms of therapy is that Hellerwork concentrates more on relieving underlying mental and emotional problems than on physical misalignments. To pursue this approach, the therapist questions the patient throughout the treatment to try to uncover underlying emotional and psychological traumas and conflicts.

In the USA, Hellerwork is thought to be particularly successful in treating people who are suffering severe emotional trauma, such as those involved in accidents and disasters, or victims of violent crime.

WATSU

Watsu is a form of water therapy based on the Eastern massage known as shiatsu. In shiatsu, the therapist uses fingers, thumbs, hands, arms, elbows and even the knees and feet to free blockages in the flow of energy through the body's energy pathways. In Watsu, a similar form of massage and manipulation is carried out while the subject floats in a warm pool. Being immersed in warm water takes the pressure off the patient's musculoskeletal system, particularly the spine and joints, making it easier for the therapist to stretch and realign the muscles and connective tissue.

Watsu aims to release stress, ease muscle tension and physical aches and pains, and to heal the spirit, as well as the mind and body. It was devised by Harold Dull, an American poet, who believed it would be beneficial to unite the healing arts of shiatsu and acupressure with the therapeutic effects of warm water. The combination of massage, manipulation and water therapy is said to strengthen blood circulation, the lymphatic system and immune response, and ease digestive and breathing problems. It is believed to relieve psychological problems such as stress, insomnia, anxiety and even addictions. It has also been used to aid the mobility of physically and mentally disabled people.

CHAPTER 3

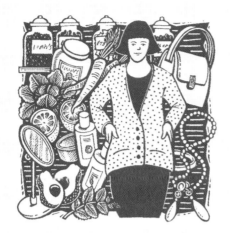

LIFESTYLE AND YOUR SHAPE

Making sure your body is fuelled for exercise through a balanced, high-carbohydrate diet will improve your health and help you to reach your shaping-up goal. In the meantime, there is a lot you can do to enhance your appearance by taking care of your skin and focusing on clothes that work with your shape and not against it.

HEALTHY EATING FOR A BETTER SHAPE

A well-balanced diet is the starting point of any shaping-up regime. It should provide the fuel you need for exercise and all the nutrients your body needs for good health.

People are often surprised to discover that, on taking up a regular exercise programme, they eat more food than previously. Because of increased appetite it can be tempting and all too easy to increase fat intake, but it is a far healthier course to increase other kinds of food, in particular carbohydrates which provide the energy for increased physical activity.

An exercise diet should not leave you feeling deprived or hungry but it is important to bring some discipline and planning into your eating routine. You will be able to have some treats – just less often. It is not just a question of the foods you eat but also when you eat them. It is important to eat at regular intervals throughout the day; skipping meals or unnecessary nibbling should become habits of the past.

When planning your exercise diet it may help to divide food into five main groups – starchy foods, such as pasta, potatoes, bread and rice; fruit and vegetables; high-protein foods, such as meat, fish and pulses; dairy products; and fatty or sugary foods.

Aim to eat higher proportions of carbohydrate, in the form of starchy foods, fruit and vegetables, while reducing your consumption of high-fat and high-sugar foods. Overall calorie requirement varies from person to person. A young active adult will need a higher calorie intake than an equally active older person, for example.

By eating the right amount of foods from each food group to meet your energy needs you will also ensure that your body receives all the essential nutrients it needs, without consuming excess fat.

Foods for weight gain

Ideally, weight gain should be due to increased muscle rather than fat. To achieve this you must combine a well-balanced exercise regime with a nutritious diet that provides more energy than your body needs. However, bear in mind that you may not be genetically programmed to put on much extra weight.

It is important to have a regular eating pattern – three meals a day with healthy snacks in between, for example, mid morning, mid afternoon and mid evening. Meals should never be skipped, and if you can, try to eat bigger portions at mealtimes.

Foods for weight loss

The only way to lose weight is to consume fewer calories than your body needs for normal bodily processes and physical activity.

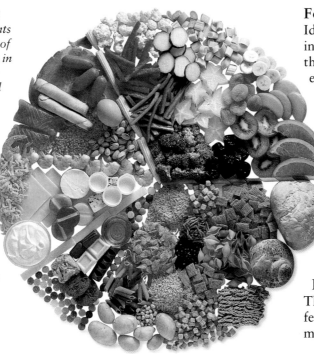

*THE RIGHT BALANCE
This piechart represents the right proportions of the main food groups in a balanced diet. Fruit and vegetables should make up one-third, while carbohydrate should make up another third. Dairy foods should be up to one-sixth, with protein almost another sixth. This leaves little room for high-fat and sugary foods which should be kept to a minimum.*

The fuel your body uses for energy comes from calories in the food you eat. Protein and carbohydrate contain 4 calories per gram while fat contains 9 calories per gram.

Most foods are a mixture of nutrients but proportions vary – foods may be mostly fat (such as butter, margarine and vegetable oils) or carbohydrate (starches and sugars) or somewhere between; no food is pure protein. As there are more calories per gram in fat than in carbohydrate and protein, high-fat foods contain the most calories. To lose weight it makes sense to cut back on the calorie-dense fatty foods and go for the less calorie-dense carbohydrate foods.

Alcohol can be used by the body for energy, but as it is a toxin it will be used in preference to fat, meaning more fat consumed will be stored, under the skin and around your internal organs.

Foods for exercise

Given that people who exercise regularly have an increased demand for energy, and that fat provides more than twice the number of calories as carbohydrate or protein on a weight for weight basis, you might be forgiven for thinking that fat is the most important component of an exercise diet. Fat does provide a good source of fuel but as we have an almost unlimited storage capacity, there is never any risk of running out and certainly no need to stock up. An excess of fat, on the other hand, can adversely affect the body's capacity for speed, strength and endurance as it simply represents 'dead' weight.

The limiting factor for sustaining peak performance during exercise is the amount of carbohydrate – in the form of glucose and glycogen – that the body has in store. To gain muscle you need to make carbohydrate the principle energy source in your diet. This will enable you to sustain an exercise programme that will stimulate muscle growth.

Protein and muscle building

Some exercisers believe that building muscle mass and maintaining strength requires a high protein intake. However, simply eating large amounts of dietary protein in any form does not increase muscle size. Only regular resistance exercise and a good all-round diet will do that.

continued on page 56

THE IMPORTANCE OF CALCIUM

Calcium is essential for healthy bones. Most bones begin in the embryo as cartilage and are gradually replaced by hard bone. This process, known as ossification, spans from about the seventh week of pregnancy, throughout childhood and into adulthood, with maximum bone mass occurring around age 30. From around 35, bone density gradually decreases and in old age thinning can result in conditions such as osteoporosis (see page 25). Women are advised to increase their calcium intake around the time of the menopause as an increased loss of bone density is common at this time.

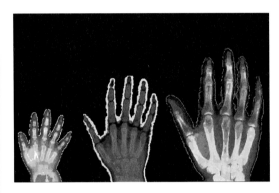

BONE GROWTH
These hand x-rays, at 30 months (left), 6 years (middle) and 19 years (right) show the hardening of bone in progress. Notice how the space between bones lessens as more cartilage ossifies.

CALCIUM CONTENT IN TYPICAL FOODS

The current UK daily calcium recommendation is 700 mg. This is easily obtainable from a balanced diet as this chart showing contents in everyday foods demonstrates.

TYPE OF FOOD	mg PER 100 g	mg PER PORTION
FISH		
Pilchards (canned in tom. sauce)	250	415 mg per 165 g portion
Salmon (canned)	300	375 mg per 125 g portion
Sardines (canned in tom. sauce)	430	430 mg per 100 g portion
DAIRY PRODUCTS		
Milk	120	240 mg per 200 ml glass
Cheese (Edam)	800	200 mg per 25 g portion
Yoghurt (low-fat)	190	260 mg per 140 g portion
VEGETABLES		
Spinach	160	160 mg per 100 g portion
Curly kale	150	150 mg per 100 g portion
Parsnip	50	50 mg per 100 g portion
Chickpeas	43	43 mg per 100 g portion
Spring greens	75	75 mg per 100 g portion
BREAD		
White bread	110	110 mg per 3 slices
Brown bread	100	100 mg per 3 slices
Wholemeal bread	54	54 mg per 3 slices

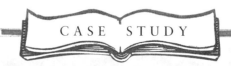
The Fatigued Gym-goer

It is all too easy to get the balance of exercise and diet wrong, particularly when the main reason for working out is to lose weight. It can be tempting to snack at the wrong times of the day and not to refuel after a work-out, especially as your appetite can be suppressed by exercise. Unfortunately this can lead to fatigue and often surprisingly little in the way of weight loss.

Anna is 33 years old, married to Roger, an advertising executive, and they have two children. Thomas is 5 years old, very boisterous and seems to manage on very little sleep. Laura is 3 years old and has become very clingy since starting at nursery. Roger's pressured work life means that the care of the children is falling solely on Anna's shoulders.

Anna has recently joined a gym, determined to lose weight before her birthday in two months' time. She decided that a combination of work-outs and strict dieting would be the answer. The easiest time to exercise seemed to be while Laura was at nursery but Anna often arrives at the gym already exhausted. Her workout, devised by the gym instructor, takes 70 minutes starting after a warm-up with 40 minutes of aerobic machine work, followed by 20 minutes using weights and a cool-down.

Anna tries to have breakfast cereal with the children but often manages nothing more than a cup of tea. While Laura has her lunch, Anna grabs a sandwich or eats whatever leftovers there may be in the fridge. The afternoon is spent playing with Laura before collecting Thomas. The children have an early tea and Anna, who is starving by now, picks at what they are having and finishes off what they leave. She doesn't think this amounts to very much in the way of calories. The next few hours are quite chaotic as Anna prepares supper for Roger and herself, and gets the children ready for bed. When Roger gets home, supper is ready but Anna is too exhausted to eat much.

What really puzzles Anna is that for all her activity, her weight is not going down very much. She feels very tempted to quit the gym – at least she feels she won't be so tired.

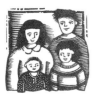

FAMILY
Young children can be very demanding on their parents' time and this can be particularly wearing when one parent is doing the bulk of the caring.

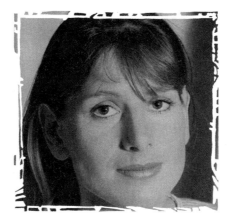

HEALTH
It is important that your body receives all the vitamins and minerals it needs from a healthy, balanced diet. Constant fatigue may be a sign of a health problem and should be checked out by a doctor.

DIET
It is easy to neglect your diet when you have a hectic lifestyle. Snacking can easily lead to overdoing fat and sugar intake and a lack of essential nutrients such as calcium and iron.

EXERCISE
Weight loss can be achieved gradually by combining exercise with a sensible weight-loss diet. Overdoing the exercise can unfortunately be counterproductive and lead to fatigue.

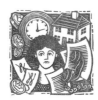

STRESS
Setting unrealistic goals can lead to increased levels of stress and subsequent irritability. Children react to this, raising stress levels further.

WHAT SHOULD ANNA DO?

Anna has set herself unrealistic targets both in her weight loss and her exercise programme. To achieve a shaping-up goal and retain it, changes in diet and exercise need to be permanent and take into consideration existing pressures – such as work and family. Anna needs to discuss her situation and requirements with the gym instructor so they can devise a more suitable exercise plan in terms of how often and how hard she is working out.

Anna's diet is very haphazard and almost certainly contains more calories than she realises. By eating very little or nothing at breakfast Anna is not fuelling her body for exercise – similarly, by skipping eating after exercise and eating little at lunchtime she is missing out on the best time to refuel her body. By waiting, she is also more likely to reach for unhealthy snacks. It could very well be that part of the tiredness is due to insufficient iron in the diet. Iron deficiency anaemia is common in women of childbearing age. It might be worth Anna going to her doctor just to make sure she is not anaemic. At the same time she could get her weight checked and take advice as to how much weight she actually needs to lose. Many women strive for a body weight which is actually below that recommended for their height.

Action Plan

FAMILY
Talk to the nursery teacher about Laura's clinginess. Ask Roger to help with the children – perhaps he could look after the children first thing in the morning or do the bedtime routine at the weekend.

DIET
Write down all food and drink consumed in a diary to see how much is actually being eaten. Make an effort to eat breakfast every day and increase carbohydrate intake at lunchtime. Refuel with carbohydrate after exercise.

EXERCISE
Speak to the gym instructor and get the programme changed to an easier one. Reduce the number of gym sessions to a manageable level.

STRESS
Assess whether weight loss is necessary by calculating BMI and draw up a workable weight-control plan. Make time in the day to relax.

HEALTH
Make an appointment to see the doctor to discuss constant fatigue and possibility of anaemia. Also ask for advice on possible diet improvements and a recommendation on ideal weight for height.

HOW THINGS TURNED OUT FOR ANNA

Anna talked to her gym instructor who reduced the intensity of her programme. As the rest of her life was quite active, he decided she would get sufficient benefit from working out twice a week. She also went to see her doctor who told her that she was not anaemic but her blood haemoglobin level could be better. The doctor recommended including more iron-rich foods in her diet and having orange juice with her breakfast rather than tea (the tannins in tea hinder iron absorption whereas vitamin C aids it). Her doctor also suggested that Anna was exaggerating her weight problem and losing a stone (6.35 kg) would actually make her underweight.

Anna followed her new gym programme and found it more enjoyable. She also realised through her food diary why she had not lost any weight. Her eating habits are now much better and she feels that her increased energy levels are in part due to her new regular eating pattern. She never misses breakfast and eats a well-planned lunch to sustain her during the day. Roger was not aware of how demanding the children had become and they drew up a plan to allow Anna some time off. As a result Anna's fatigue is greatly reduced and she is now enjoying life much more. Interestingly, Laura is back to her old sociable self too.

Calories and kilocalories

The energy in the foods you eat is measured in units called calories, which is the energy needed to raise the temperature of one millilitre of water by 1°C. To overcome the problem of counting in such small units, health and nutrition professionals usually speak in terms of kilocalories or Calories (capital 'C') which equal 1000 calories and are often abbreviated as kcal or Cal. Another term often used is the kilojoule, which is an even smaller unit of calories: 4.18 kilojoules equals one calorie.

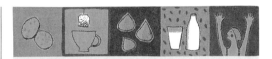

SUPER SHAPER

Chestnuts are an ideal component of a diet geared towards exercise as they are high in energy and low in calories. They have about four times the carbohydrate content of other nuts but only 5–10 per cent of the fat. They are also good sources of vitamins E and B6 and minerals iron, manganese, magnesium and potassium. Chestnuts can be eaten raw but have a slightly bitter flavour. They taste sweeter when cooked and can be roasted or baked. They are delicious when served with green vegetables, such as Brussels sprouts, and can be puréed as a stuffing, ground up and made into biscuits, or sweetened for use in desserts.

Those who exercise on a regular basis need more protein than those who do not exercise but this increased requirement is easily met by the normal diet and there is no need to take a protein supplement. The best way to maintain an adequate protein intake is to eat a wide variety of foods.

Foods for healthy bones

During youth and adulthood, bones become stronger by accumulating calcium (see page 53). This continues until around 30 years of age, when peak bone mass is reached. After this a slow decline in bone mass in men and women occurs as more calcium is lost than is gained through the diet.

This loss accelerates in women after the menopause when the level of the female hormone oestrogen, which maintains bone mass, starts to fall. Reduced bone mass can lead to osteoporosis, a brittle-bone condition causing stooped posture, reduced height, and increased risk of bone fractures. The condition, thought to be in part due to genetic factors, currently affects one in four postmenopausal women and one in twelve men. The incidence is rising but there is strong evidence that the rate of post-menopausal bone loss can be reduced by diet and exercise.

To maximise peak bone mass and slow the rate of bone loss it is important that throughout your life you regularly exercise, consume adequate amounts of vitamin D, and ensure a good intake of calcium.

Spacing your meals

Your diet needs to be organised to ensure you get all the nutrients needed in the right amounts and at the right times. Plan your meals each day, taking note of the following points to ensure that you maximise your nutrient intake over the day.

Eat meals and snacks at regular intervals, but take care not to increase your overall food intake – the aim is to eat less at each meal but more often; this helps to stabilise blood glucose and insulin levels, controls blood cholesterol and reduces the risk of storing excess fat.

Each time you eat, you increase your metabolic rate (the energy you need just to keep your body functioning) because of the extra demands of digesting, absorbing, transporting and metabolising the food. This can help the energy balance. Spacing your meals and snacks so that you can eat soon after exercise will speed recovery by helping to replace the stores of glycogen that have been used during the session.

What to eat before, during and after an exercise session

Pre-exercise carbohydrate is useful for anyone who works their body extremely hard, especially athletes in training. It does not trigger a surge of insulin leading to a low blood sugar level, as some people fear, but helps you to maintain higher blood sugar levels, which delays fatigue. It can also improve endurance allowing you to train harder for longer. A banana, dried fruit, jam sandwich or a sports drink consumed 5–30 minutes before training is beneficial if a long hard exercise session is being undertaken.

Having carbohydrate during your exercise session may help to increase muscle strength and size and delay fatigue but again this depends on how long and hard you are

DID YOU KNOW?
Even in the leanest of athletes there is never any shortage of fat available for fuel. For example, a 70 kg (11 stone) male athlete with a body fat of just 10 per cent has a fat store equivalent to 60 000 kcals.

exercising. Carbohydrate (food or drink) must be consumed early in the session if you are to reap any rewards. Drinking is the easiest method of consuming carbohydrate during exercise and has a twofold benefit as the fluids also help to prevent dehydration. If you prefer to eat, choose those foods recommended for pre-exercise fuelling.

It is important to consume carbohydrate soon after exercise as the body's stores of glycogen from carbohydrate is replenished most efficiently in the first one to two hours after a training session. If you don't refuel properly (if you miss a meal or eat a high-fat meal) you may feel tired the next day and sluggish during your next exercise session as your muscles have not fully refilled their glycogen stores.

Appetite is often suppressed after exercise but most people feel thirsty; sports drinks which include carbohydrate are a good choice. If you do eat after exercise choose bananas, dried fruit, cereal bars or bread, followed two to four hours later by a high-carbohydrate meal.

High-energy sports drinks

Specially formulated sports drinks are becoming more and more popular but it is important to have the right drink at the right time. Research shows that isotonic and hypotonic drinks, which contain 2–8 per cent carbohydrate (such as glucose, sucrose, maltodextrin or glucose polymer) and some sodium, are absorbed faster than water alone and can therefore help to prevent you getting dehydrated during an exercise session. The carbohydrate in the drink will top up your fuel reserves.

Depletion of glycogen stores and dehydration are the main causes of fatigue so it is important to prevent this. These drinks are therefore very suitable before, during and immediately after an exercise session when rehydration is important.

Hypertonic drinks have a higher carbohydrate content (over 10 per cent) but are not as effective at rehydrating as the fluid takes longer to enter the bloodstream. Such drinks should be saved for refuelling or when rehydration is not the priority.

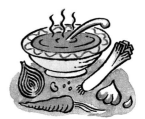

SOUP YOURSELF UP
A variety of warming soups can be made ahead and frozen so that you have a nutritious, high-carbohydrate meal in a flash. Ideal ingredients include lentils, barley, split peas and fresh vegetables.

STOCKING FOODS FOR POWER SNACKS

High-energy snacks and meals can be useful for topping up energy levels a couple of hours before an exercise session or an hour or two after exercise when the body's refuelling is at its most efficient. The aim is to eat or drink something that is predominantly made up of carbohydrates that are rapidly digested and absorbed by the body but low in fat. Make a list of all the foods you like that you can use to quickly make a nutritious high-carbohydrate meal. Keep your kitchen stocked with these food items. Perishables will need replacing each time you go shopping – check your cupboards to see if you are low on any other items.

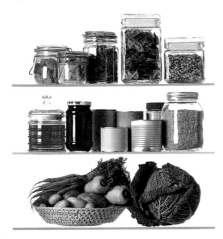

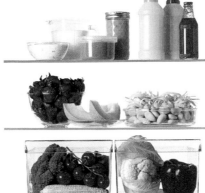

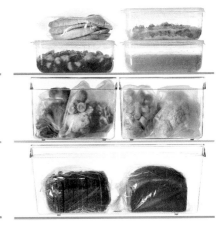

IN THE CUPBOARD
Bread, breakfast cereals, pasta, rice, fresh vegetables, dried fruit, tinned tomatoes, beans, sweetcorn and fish (in brine or water), peanut butter, honey, pasta sauces and tinned soups.

IN THE FRIDGE
Low-fat yoghurts, low-fat cheese, milk (skimmed or semi-skimmed), fresh fruit juices, fresh soup, fresh pasta, fruit and vegetables such as strawberries, melon, tomatoes and sweetcorn.

IN THE FREEZER
Extra bread, rolls, pitta bread, pizza bases, fruit buns, lean mince, chicken or turkey fillets, fish steaks, frozen vegetables and preprepared meals such as casseroles and soups.

SUPPLEMENTS – DO THEY WORK?

There is no shortage of supplements directed at the exercising public, but it is important to know whether dietary aids taken as part of a shaping-up regime have any proven benefits.

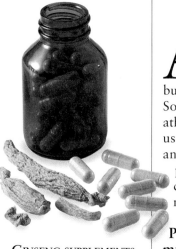

GINSENG SUPPLEMENTS
Many people, including athletes, take ginseng supplements to boost their energy levels. But studies carried out in 1996 and 1997 in the US involving groups of people of average fitness showed no improvement in their metabolism or exercise performance while they were taking ginseng supplements. The studies were only conducted over periods of two to three months, however, so it may be that the benefits of ginseng only arise from long-term use.

A wide range of dietary supplements are available that claim to enhance exercise performance, boost muscle building, reduce fat and aid general health. Some are targeted primarily at the serious athlete, but many people may be tempted to use supplements as part of a general diet and exercise programme. While some supplements can be beneficial in certain cases, others have little proven effect and may even be harmful.

Protein supplements for muscle building

A well-balanced diet alone will easily supply all the protein you need and there is no need to use protein supplements. Increasing your daily protein intake will not automatically encourage any increase in muscle mass – indeed there are no special foods that directly boost strength or muscle size.

Excess protein is eliminated by the kidneys and there has been some concern that this may lead to dehydration as more water is needed to get rid of the excess. However, with healthy kidneys and a good fluid intake, harmful effects are unlikely. Protein beyond that eliminated by the kidneys is either burned as energy or stored as fat.

Some high-protein diets are associated with high fat intakes, and this could increase the risk of heart disease. Too much protein in the diet may also lead to reduced intake of carbohydrate, which in turn may lead to a state of chronic fatigue. This will exacerbate the problem of excess protein because it will limit the amount of exercise that can be performed, so that even less dietary protein is converted into muscle. Finally, a high protein intake may lead to an increased loss of calcium from the body.

Vitamins and minerals

Vitamins have long been of interest to regular exercisers, many believing that training can be improved by consuming vitamins in larger amounts than available in a normal diet. Vitamins and minerals do have an important role in the efficient functioning of the body, but taking too much of any vitamin cannot improve performance and could be harmful.

Although a balanced diet should provide the body with all the nutrients it requires, particular people may benefit from vitamin supplements. For example, it is recommended that some athletes take iron supplements in order to keep their energy levels to a maximum. Iron is an important constituent of the blood pigment found in muscles and is a participant in energy-producing reactions of the body. Older people, and those with gastrointestinal disorders, who have difficulty in obtaining sufficient nutrients from their diet, may also benefit from taking supplements.

Fat mobilising supplements

Some substances, sold as 'fat mobilisers', claim to break up fat and assist its removal from the body but at present, no scientific evidence can back this up. The only proven way to 'mobilise' fat is to combine aerobic exercise with a low-fat diet.

One substance sold as a fat mobilising agent is carnitine, which is necessary for the transport of fats into the mitochondria – microscopic structures that act as the powerhouse of each body cell (see box, right). The theory that carnitine can push more fats across to be used as fuel is not supported. Inositol is another supposed fat mobiliser. But its value as a supplement is doubtful as

FAT BURNERS IN THE MUSCLE CELLS

Some food supplements are claimed to speed the rate at which fat passes into tiny powerhouses called mitochondria, found in all cells, to be burnt as energy. But this has not been scientifically proven. Mitochondria break down fatty acids and other food molecules to release energy. They are most numerous in highly active cells such as muscle cells, or fibres. The inner membrane of the mitochondria is folded to form shelves (cristae). The spaces between the cristae contain the enzymes needed to break down fatty acids.

ENERGY CONVERSION
Muscle cells used in aerobic activities contain thousands of mitochondria. Mitochondria use oxygen to convert fat into muscle energy.

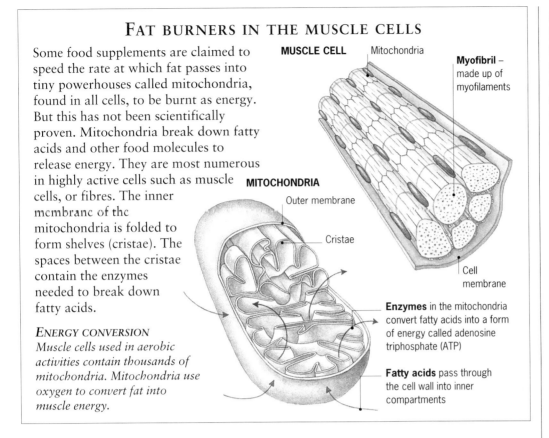

MUSCLE CELL Mitochondria

Myofibril – made up of myofilaments

MITOCHONDRIA

Outer membrane

Cristae

Cell membrane

Enzymes in the mitochondria convert fatty acids into a form of energy called adenosine triphosphate (ATP)

Fatty acids pass through the cell wall into inner compartments

Steroid abuse
In 1968 the Olympic Games banned the use of performance-enhancing drugs such as anabolic steroids and introduced drug testing. In 1970 the Commonwealth Games followed suit greeted by protests from the Eastern bloc. It is now known that many athletes, under extreme pressure to succeed, have used performance enhancing drugs, despite being linked to over 70 health damaging side effects. Anabolic steroids are still used by some athletes during training, but the International Olympic Committee now claim they can detect illegal drug use as far back as eight weeks.

it can be made in the body and it is not proven to function as a fat mobiliser. It is similar for lecithin, which emulsifies fats and aids digestion, but does not aid fat loss.

Body-building chemicals

Male hormones, called androgens, belong to a group of chemicals called 'steroids' because they have a ring-shaped, or steroid, atomic structure. Androgens – testosterone in particular – cause a variety of effects. They are mainly responsible for the development of male sexual traits in puberty – their 'androgenic' effect – and also play a part in sexual libido.

Androgens are also 'anabolic' hormones, so stimulate muscle growth and development. Anabolic steroids are synthetic drugs that have a similar effect to androgens. They have many undesirable physical and psychological side effects, which can damage health and may even be life threatening. These include acne, hair loss, oily skin, deepening of the voice, abnormal hair growth on the face and body, masculinisation in women, breast enlargement in males, and reduced sperm production. They can also cause personality changes, liver damage and heart disease.

Anabolic steroids should not be confused with corticosteroid drugs, sometimes called steroids, which are used to treat inflammatory conditions and other disorders.

A number of supplements, mainly made from plant extracts, also claim to boost the body's production of testosterone and so boost muscle mass. These claims are unsupported. Such supplements include gamma oryzanol, a plant sterol derived from rice bran oil, smilax and yohimbine.

VITAMIN LOADING AND MEGADOSES

When vitamins are taken in very large amounts – known as megadoses – they no longer function as vitamins but as drugs with medicinal actions. Evidence for the therapeutic effects of megadosing is still highly controversial.

The vitamins that have the most toxic effects when taken in excess are the fat soluble kinds A, D and, to a lesser extent, E and K, which are easily stored in the body and can build up to harmful levels. The water soluble vitamin B complex and C are thought to be less harmful because it is believed that any excess is excreted by the body. However, some B vitamins are believed to lead to nerve disorders when taken in excess, and too much vitamin C can cause diarrhoea and may lead to kidney stones in susceptible people.

TONING UP YOUR SKIN

Although a daily regime of cleansing and moisturising goes a long way towards a healthy complexion, the condition of your skin is also a reflection of your lifestyle and diet.

The skin is the largest organ of the body, and is the first line of defence in protecting the internal organs and muscles of the body from damage and disease. It regulates your body's temperature, increasing sweating if you get too hot and erecting the hair follicles or causing goose pimples if you get cold. It is important for everyone, regardless of age, sex or race, to look after their skin. The first step is to feed the skin from the inside out by eating a healthy, balanced diet rich in vitamins. A routine of cleansing, exfoliating, toning and moisturising is important not only for women but also for men. In addition, certain lifestyle factors, such as smoking and exposure to the sun, should be avoided in order to minimise damage to the skin.

THE STRUCTURE OF SKIN

The skin is made up of two main layers, the epidermis and the dermis, with an underlying layer of subcutaneous tissue, which is mostly adipose tissue (fat).

The epidermis is the skin's protective layer. It contains rapidly dividing basal cells made up of a hard substance called keratin. New cells travel to the surface of the epidermis and die, forming a tough outer coating. As these cells wear away they are replaced by new ones. Some cells produce the pigment melanin which determines skin colour – the more of these cells that are present, the darker the natural skin colour.

The dermis is made up of connective tissue such as collagen and elastin, which, together with subcutaneous fat, are responsible for the skin's shape and elasticity. This layer houses hair follicles, sweat glands, and sebaceous glands, which produce the oily substance sebum. The dermis also houses blood and lymph vessels, which provide nutrients and remove wastes, and the skin's sensory nerve endings.

SKIN TYPES

Sebum is the skin's natural lubricant, keeping your hair and skin moisturised. If not enough is produced it causes dry skin, while overproduction leads to oily skin. Knowing

HOW SPOTS DEVELOP

Each hair follicle contains a sebaceous gland producing sebum, your body's own moisturiser, keeping hair and skin supple. If excess sebum is produced (such as at puberty), it can clog the opening to the hair follicle, trapping bacteria inside. This causes the hair to die and a spot to form. Keep your pores clear with regular cleansing.

NORMAL HAIR FOLLICLE
Excess sebum is produced by the sebaceous gland and flows to the surface.

Hair follicle

Sebum

Sebaceous gland

Hair bulb

Adipose tissue

Trapped sebum

Plug

SPOT FORMS
Sebum and dead cells plug the opening to the pore, trapping bacteria inside and causing a spot to form.

your skin type will help you to look after it and avoid skin irritations and premature ageing.

Dry skin This type of skin tends to have a fine, papery or chalky texture which chaps easily and feels tight after washing. Regular moisturising is important as the sebaceous glands do not produce enough oil to lubricate it. Sebum declines with age so it is even more important to moisturise the skin in later life.

Oily skin Usually shiny and slightly greasy, this type of skin often gives a sallow complexion with open pores. Because of the overproduction of sebum, the pores get clogged and so spots and blackheads are common. Teenagers often have oily skin caused by excess production of sex hormones. Most people have less spots as they age because the level of sebum produced declines. However, some people have oily skin throughout their lives. There is some good news for these people – oily skin stays free of wrinkles for longer than any other skin type. Regular cleansing is important to keep the pores clear.

Combination skin People of this skin type have both dry and oily patches. The oily patches tend to be the T-shaped area of the forehead, nose and chin, while the cheeks are dry. Oily skin types often develop combination skin with age. Light moisturising and the use of toning agents on oily areas keeps skin clear.

Normal skin This skin has a soft, supple texture and is clear of blemishes, with no dry or oily patches. It can become dry with age and is more likely to wrinkle. Light moisturising after washing is all that is needed for this type of skin, until dryness becomes more marked with age when more thorough moisturising will be necessary.

EATING FOR HEALTHY SKIN

Eating a varied diet that includes fruit, vegetables, seeds and grains is good for your body and this is reflected in the condition of your skin. For a truly healthy skin, your skin care regime has to start from within.

The first step towards healthy skin is to drink lots of liquid, 6–8 glasses of water or fruit juice a day, to restore the body's fluid levels and flush toxins out of the system, so improving the complexion. Skin also needs a variety of vitamins and minerals which purify the

blood and keep the complexion clear. The most important are the antioxidant vitamins A, C and E, beta carotene, and the mineral selenium. Antioxidants combat harmful free radicals, which are unstable molecules produced as a part of normal bodily processes, by pollution, sunlight and cigarettes. They attack the cells causing tissue damage and wrinkles. Antioxidants can be obtained from various sources including fresh fruits, especially citrus fruits and berries, and from brightly coloured or green, leafy vegetables.

INDIVIDUAL SUMMER PUDDINGS

This recipe, packed with delicious berry fruits, is an excellent source of antioxidants which feed your skin from the inside out.

about 15 slices medium-sliced white bread, crusts removed
about 700 g/1½ lb mixed berry fruits such as blackberries, raspberries, strawberries, blueberries and cherries
1 tbsp sugar
half-fat crème fraîche to serve
mint sprigs to decorate

■ Line six mini pudding bowls (6 fl oz capacity) with the bread slices, cutting them to fit where necessary – do not overlap (reserve some bread slices to make the pudding lids).
■ Hull and halve the strawberries. Remove stalks from other berries and wash.

■ Gently heat blueberries and cherries (if using) in a saucepan with 1 tbsp sugar and 5 tbsp water over low heat. Cook, stirring, until fruit is tender. Remove from heat and add rest of the fruit, stirring gently to mix.
■ Spoon the fruit and most of the juice equally into the bread-lined bowls (reserve a little juice for serving). Make a lid for each pudding with the reserved bread slices. Place the filled bowls on a tray in the refrigerator to catch any overflowing juices. Put a weighted saucer over the top of each to keep the 'lids' in place.
■ Remove the weighted saucers and invert the puddings onto six serving plates. Spoon the reserved juices over the top, garnish with mint sprigs and serve with a dollop of crème fraîche.
Serves 6

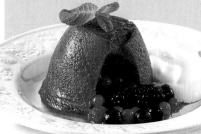

Skin Cleansers

Making your own skin cleansers from easily obtainable natural products can save you money and also offer other benefits. For example, you will know that there are no additives that may irritate sensitive skin and that it hasn't been tested on animals.

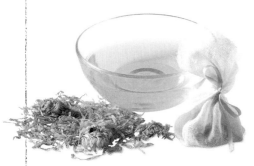

HERBAL INFUSION
If you prefer, use a herbal infusion instead of the water in the cleanser below. Wrap 2 tablespoons of a dried herb such as marigold in muslin, pour over boiling water, cover and infuse for 10 minutes.

The natural substances in these cleansers offer special properties that benefit particular skin types. For example, papaya has a natural fruit acid (AHA) content that leaves the skin looking smoother, and papain, an enzyme in papaya, helps digest protein and remove dead skin cells. These properties help to boost the complexion and dry out spots. Take care to avoid the skin around the eyes when applying cleanser. As long as they don't include fresh ingredients, homemade cleansers will keep for about a month in an airtight container in the fridge.

BEESWAX AND ALMOND CLEANSING CREAM

This soft, fluffy cream is suitable for most skin types. Wax is flammable so it needs to be heated slowly. The best way to do this is to use a water bath, or *bain marie* (a bowl set over boiling water). This heats the ingredients by steam rather than direct heat.

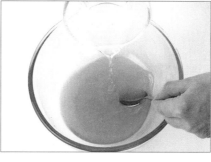

1 *Heat 25 g (1 oz) beeswax and 160 ml almond oil in a water bath until the wax melts. In another water bath, heat 150 ml (5 fl oz) water and 2.5 ml (½ tsp) borax to the same temperature.*

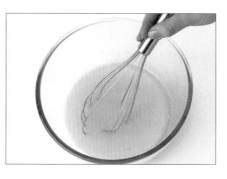

2 *Remove both bowls from the heat and, stirring constantly, pour the water and borax mixture into the beeswax mixture. Continue to stir until the cream thickens and starts to cool.*

3 *Add about 10 drops of chosen essential oils (see below), beat the cream until cooled and spoon into a dark coloured glass jar. Apply with circular movements, using clean fingertips or a piece of cotton wool. After about 30 seconds, remove with a tissue or dampened cotton wool.*
Essential oils: dry skin - jasmine, rose, lavender; oily skin - geranium, bergamot, rosemary; sensitive skin - camomile.

PAPAYA CLEANSER FOR PROBLEM SKIN

Cut a well-ripened papaya in half and remove the seeds. Scoop out the flesh and whizz in a blender until a smooth consistency. Stroke the papaya over the face using gentle, circular movements. Leave for a few minutes and then wipe off with a tissue and rinse with plenty of warm water.

GRAPEFRUIT CLEANSER FOR OILY SKIN

This cleanser is ideal if you enjoy grapefruit for breakfast. After eating your grapefruit cut the empty shell into sections. Rub the white fleshy side in a circular action all over your face. Leave it a few minutes then rinse off with warm water and pat dry. Your skin will feel silky smooth.

Some foods should be avoided or consumed in moderation because they have a harmful effect on the skin. Excess fats, for example, cause an overproduction of free radicals in the body. They can also harm the lymph system, which has an important role to play in detoxifying the skin.

Stimulants such as tea, coffee and alcohol increase fluid loss from the body, through increased sweating and urination, leading to dehydration. This reduces the skin's capacity to receive nutrients and remove toxins. Alcohol also depletes the body of B and C vitamins, causing wrinkles and poor skin tone. Heavy alcohol consumption leads to facial flushing, due to widening of small blood vessels just below the surface of the skin, and can become permanent.

Smoked, barbecued and processed foods and cigarettes also increase levels of free radicals and reduce antioxidants in the body. Among other problems, this causes premature skin ageing. Antioxidant supplements, especially vitamin C and E, can help to alleviate this but are no alternative to giving up smoking, moderating alcohol intake and having a healthy and varied diet.

PREVENTING SKIN DAMAGE

Many of the threats to a healthy skin come from the environment, both indoors and out. Excess sunlight, pollution, dry atmospheres, wind and rain, heat and cold, and cigarette smoke, can all damage the skin.

Ultraviolet rays from the sun can penetrate the dermis and break down collagen, even in winter, causing skin sagging and premature wrinkles. Although a little exposure helps the body to produce vitamin D, sunlight that is strong enough to tan the skin, and cause peeling, can age the skin prematurely. To keep a youthful complexion for longer, it is advisable to protect the skin from bright sunlight. Apply a low factor sunscreen (5–10) in winter and a high factor (15 plus) in summer.

After sunlight, cigarette smoke has the most damaging effect on the skin. Smokers have far more wrinkles than nonsmokers and often have pale, grey or sallow complexions. The skin is also thicker and may have broken veins. Smoking also depletes vitamin C levels in the body, so skin damage heals at a slower rate. Eating foods rich in vitamin C or taking a supplement can help but more importantly smoking's effect on the skin is yet another reason, along with increased well-being and reduced risk of major diseases, for giving up altogether.

Central heating and air conditioning produce an arid atmosphere that quickly dries the skin. You can counteract this by using humidifiers, or placing a bowl of water by a radiator, to add moisture to the air. Cold winds also dry the skin so use moisturiser regularly to compensate. Sudden changes in temperature – going straight out into the cold from a warm room, for example – can cause delicate blood vessels in the skin to burst resulting in thread veins (spider naevi) on the cheeks and nose. To avoid this, lower the room temperature or move to a cooler room to give your body more time to adjust before going outside.

THE AGEING PROCESS

Skin has an in-built biological clock in its cells. This determines how and when it will age. This natural, inevitable process varies for each of us, depending on our genetic inheritance. Look at your parents to see how their skin has aged and you will get a good idea of what will happen to you.

From the age of about 30 years, the plump, unwrinkled skin of youth begins to change. The cells do not renew themselves so readily and the other functions of the skin, such as oil production, begin to slow down. At the same time, the skin loses its flexibility due to reduced collagen production. With natural ageing, the skin's outer layer becomes thinner, making it less resistant to damage. It also loses its elasticity and wrinkles begin to appear.

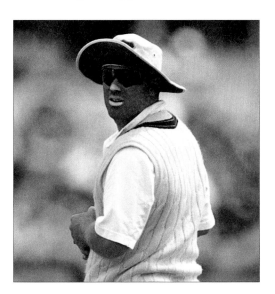

SPORT AND SKIN CARE
Sensible sun precautions, shown here by Australian cricketer, Shane Warne, include a hat to keep the sun off the face and the back of the neck, sunglasses to protect the eyes and total sunblock on sensitive areas such as the nose and lips. For sport, use waterproof sun cream as sweat from exertion can quickly wash other creams away. Reapply cream regularly.

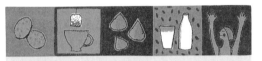

SUPER SHAPER

Cleopatra knew a good beauty product when she bathed in it – milk protein has the same effect on skin as when we drink it. It builds, repairs and reconditions. Milk has a lactic acid base that can actually reinforce the skin's natural acid mantle which protects against the harmful effects of bacteria, alcohol, smoke, sun and wind, and helps to maintain the skin's pH balance. Milk is becoming an increasingly popular ingredient for beauty products including milk baths, milk soap bars and milk shampoo. In fact, milk can be used straight from the fridge as a cleanser, nourishing the skin as you use it.

As well as genetic factors and natural ageing, your skin is subjected to a number of damaging forces – sunlight, wind and excessive heat and cold. Environmental pollution such as car exhaust fumes, background radiation and other toxic emissions can also take their toll. Sometimes the skin displays an allergic reaction to substances such as medications and cosmetics. Skin also reacts adversely to emotional stress, lack of exercise, sleep deprivation and occasionally to fluctuating hormone levels.

Exercise and skin problems

Although exercise is excellent for the skin, sometimes problems can occur. Sweat, if left on the skin, can cause bacteria to breed, causing body odour. Bacteria live on the skin's surface and when the sweat comes into contact with it, an unpleasant odour occurs. However, this odour takes a few hours to develop, so provided you wash regularly and use an antiperspirant, it should not be a problem. If you suffer from excessive sweating, you may need to see your doctor for a stronger, prescription antiperspirant.

There are other skin problems caused indirectly through exercise, the most common being fungal infections. Athlete's foot, commonly acquired at swimming pools, causes an itchy red rash and flaking skin between the toes and on the soles of the feet. The skin may crack, causing painful open sores. People with sweaty feet are more prone to athlete's foot. Topical antifungal creams and powders are available to kill the fungi or to prevent them from growing. Sometimes, for persistent cases, your doctor may prescribe antifungal tablets to be taken for about three months.

Chlorine in swimming pools can also irritate sensitive skin. There is a trend towards lowering the amount of chlorine in the water, which may help to reduce the discomfort so try to find a pool that advertises this facility. Always shower thoroughly after swimming and calm the skin down with camomile cream.

Blisters from ill-fitting sports shoes are very painful but usually clear up once the shoes are discarded and the blister has burst naturally – never burst a blister yourself.

SKIN CLEANSERS

The skin is covered with cavities where dirt, grime, oil and dead skin cells accumulate, leading to spots and blackheads. Cleansing the skin, first thing in the morning and last thing at night, removes impurities and allows the skin to breathe. There are several types to choose from.

Soap This is usually alkaline and can irritate the skin, which is the opposite – naturally slightly acidic. Some soaps include moisturisers and are not so alkaline, which makes them kinder to the skin.

Cream cleansers With a rich consistency, these contain emulsifiers to dissolve dirt particles. Rich, creamy types should be lightly massaged over the skin, while thinner types should be applied and then removed with cotton wool.

Liquid cleansers Milky or creamy, these should be lightly applied to the face and then removed with tissue or cotton wool.

DID YOU KNOW?

According to ancient Roman legend, the word 'soap' derived from Mount Sapo, a place where animals were sacrificed. Rain washed a mixture of animal fat, or tallow, and wood ashes down into the clay soil along the River Tiber. Women, who washed their clothes in the river, found that using this clay mixture made their wash cleaner.

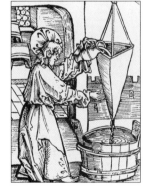

AN ANCIENT ART
This woodcut showing the making of lye, a liquid solution of potash essential for soapmaking, dates from 1514. It is not known exactly when soap was discovered but it may have been as far back as prehistoric times. The earliest known recording is of the Babylonians making soap around 2800 BC.

Making Your Own

Moisturisers

Moisturisers help your skin to recover from day-to-day damage. Using natural ingredients to make your own means that they will be fresh and any active constituents such as vitamins, minerals and essential fatty acids, will be more effective.

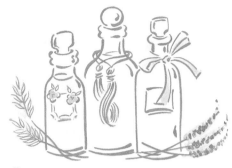

Homemade products can often be more effective than expensive shop-bought ones. Most homemade products will last about a month, but this time may be reduced to just a few days if fresh ingredients are used. As with cleanser, avoid the eye area when applying moisturiser and always test a small amount of a new product on your skin before applying large quantities, particularly if you have sensitive or allergy-prone skin.

PRESENTING HOMEMADE PRODUCTS
Select attractive, airtight glass jars or ceramic pots for your products. With some simple decoration, they will make a special gift with a personal touch.

AVOCADO AND HONEY CREAM FOR DRY OR OLDER SKINS

These skins lack moisture so choose products such as avocado that are good skin lubricants. Avocado contains plant oils that are rich in essential fatty acids – particularly linoleic acid – which are not only natural moisturisers but also strengthen the membranes that surround the skin cells. Keep this cream in the refrigerator and use within three days.

• Using a food processor, wire masher or pestle and mortar, mash half a ripe avocado until smooth and lump free. You may need to push it through a sieve to get it smooth.
• Add 1 tbsp honey or olive oil and a drop of calendula essential oil; stir until completely combined. If you have thread veins, sensitive, mature or wrinkled skin you can substitute neroli essential oil for the calendula.

PEPPERMINT AND TEA TREE CREAM FOR OILY SKIN

Oily skins do need moisturising but products with a high oil content should be avoided. This cream uses jojoba oil which closely matches the skin's own oil, sebum, making it ideal for oily skin. In addition, this cream uses tea tree oil which has an antiseptic quality and is an effective treatment for acne-prone skin.

• In a water bath over medium heat, melt together 11 g (⅓ oz) grated beeswax and 4 tsp jojoba oil. Meanwhile prepare 75 ml/3 fl oz tea using peppermint tea bags. Add ½ tsp borax into the hot tea.
• Remove the wax from the heat and slowly trickle in the tea whisking constantly with a wire or electric hand whisk, until an emulsion has formed.
• Cool slightly then blend 8 drops peppermint and 4 drops tea tree oil into the mixture, stirring to combine.

RICH CITRUS NIGHT CREAM FOR ALL SKIN TYPES

Suitable for all skin types, this cream can be easily made from everyday ingredients. Because it uses fresh ingredients it will only last about a week. Apply with clean fingers and wipe off any excess with tissue or cotton wool after about 20 minutes.

• Squeeze ½ tsp juice from a small lemon and 1 tsp juice from an orange into a medium bowl.
• Add 3 egg yolks and 1 tsp glycerine to the juice and beat with a whisk until well combined.
• Drizzle 2–3 tsp olive oil very slowly into the mixture, beating all the time, until the mixture is thick.
• Beat in 1–2 tbsp yoghurt to thin the mixture to the desired consistency.

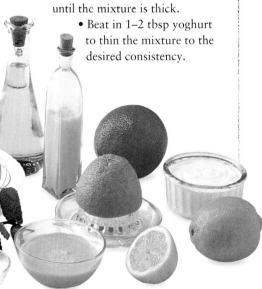

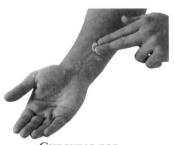

CHECKING FOR SENSITIVITY
Even if you do not think that you have sensitive skin, it is always best to test a new product, whether shop bought or homemade. Place a small amount on an area of soft sensitive skin and leave it for 5 minutes. If there is no reaction you can safely apply it more freely.

Water soluble cleansers These are applied to damp skin, massaged in and then washed off with warm water.

Gel or oil cleansers Massage these onto slightly damp skin and then rinse off with warm water. Some have antiseptic properties to help to combat spots or acne.

Body washes These are used as a substitute for soap, mainly in the shower. The wash is massaged over the skin and then rinsed off under the shower.

CLEANSERS FOR DIFFERENT SKIN TYPES

Each type of cleanser suits different kinds of skin. It is important to choose the right one for your skin type.

Soap is too astringent for dry and older skins. Instead, a richer cleanser should be used to remove make-up and daily grime, followed by a toner lotion to remove any traces of cleanser. Only rinse your face in water afterwards if you live in a soft water area. Hard water contains mineral deposits that accumulate on the skin.

A mild soap is suitable for oily and combination skins but use a cleansing lotion first to remove make-up. Medicated soaps are suitable for patches prone to spots, but avoid using them on dry areas as they can cause scaling. Mild soaps or cleansing lotions are fine for normal skins but you may need to try different types to find the most suitable kind for your skin.

MOISTURISERS

Environmental conditions and cleansing can deplete your skin of sebum so you need to replace it with moisturiser. Most daytime moisturisers include sun protection factors and soothing herbal extracts that help to combat skin irritations.

The richest moisturisers are water-based (oil-in-water emulsions) and are most suited to dry or older skins or for use during winter to guard against strong wind. Most lotions, creams and gels are water-based.

A lighter moisturiser is produced from an oil-based (water-in-oil) preparation which is more easily absorbed by the skin. This type suits normal, combination and oily skins. Most ointments are oil-based.

Night cleansing is often more rigorous in order to remove the daily accumulation of dirt and make-up, so night moisturising creams tend to be richer and are designed to

---

ALOE VERA AND COCONUT SHAVING CREAM

This shaving cream is ideal for a man's beard or for women to use on legs and underarms. The soothing properties of coconut calm the skin while the healing aloe vera gel deals with any razor nicks. Natural plant oils leave the skin silky smooth with no need to use an additional moisturiser after shaving. Store in an airtight tub and use within one month. After shaving, remove excess cream with a hot damp flannel and pat the skin dry.

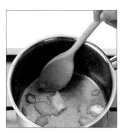 **1** *Melt 175 g (6 oz) coconut oil over low heat. When liquid, remove from heat and whisk in 2 tsp witch hazel and 50 ml (2 fl oz) almond oil.*

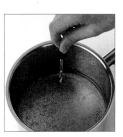 **2** *Whisk in 1 tbsp aloe vera gel until combined. Leave to cool slightly then add 8 drops lavender essential oil. Leave to set in the fridge.*

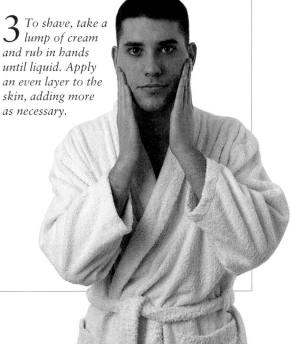 **3** *To shave, take a lump of cream and rub in hands until liquid. Apply an even layer to the skin, adding more as necessary.*

The Middle-aged Acne Sufferer

Diet and exercise should go hand in hand towards a healthy body and mind. However, too much exercise can suppress the immune system and when the diet is wrong too, this can sometimes lead to skin problems. Emotional factors affect the physical body too – if both body and mind are under stress, other physical problems can occur.

Gwen is a 44-year-old part-time dental nurse. After her divorce three years ago, she took up exercise and now attends a health club for step aerobics, gym, circuit training and tennis.

Although her complexion has always remained reasonably clear, Gwen has had occasional outbreaks of spots on her face, back and chest. Recently this has become worse. She has also developed a skin infection between her thighs and under her breasts. She has suffered athlete's foot in the past and the symptoms seem similar.

Gwen went to see her GP, who identified her fungal infection as intertrigo, and prescribed an anti-fungal cream. He recommended a retinol-based cream for her spots.

WHAT SHOULD GWEN DO?

Gwen should use the acne and anti-fungal creams as prescribed and her skin will slowly begin to improve. Eager to prevent recurrence, Gwen decided to visit a homeopath to investigate if her different skin problems are linked. After a long interview, the practitioner identified a strong emotional link between her skin outbreaks and her divorce. Gwen was finding being alone hard to deal with. Further questioning revealed that she was eating a very poor diet as she no longer always cooked an evening meal. She was also overdoing the exercise, as it fulfilled her need for company. All these factors had combined to lower her immune system, leaving her more prone to infections.

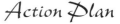

Action Plan

DIET
Establish a regular eating pattern, reduce saturated fat and sugar, and eat more fruit and vegetables, to purify the skin and boost the immune system.

EXERCISE
Temporarily reduce exercise level to allow the body to direct its energy towards strengthening the immune system.

EMOTIONAL HEALTH
Seek help from a counsellor to help solve deep-rooted emotional conflicts which may be the cause of the skin problem.

DIET
A diet low in fruit and vegetables but high in fats and sugar creates an environment for infection to thrive and suppresses the immune system.

EXERCISE
Moderate exercise can aid the immune system, but when taken to excess it can reduce the body's ability to fight infection.

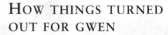

HOW THINGS TURNED OUT FOR GWEN

Gwen reduced her activities to sessions of tennis and aerobics and used the prescribed creams religiously. She began taking homeopathic tablets for her skin, wrote down some diet rules and stuck to them. She also saw a counsellor who helped her to deal with her suppressed emotions.

Gwen is feeling much more optimistic and healthier, knowing that she is dealing positively with her physical and emotional problems.

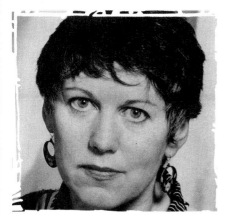

EMOTIONAL HEALTH
Activity can often be a way of avoiding emotional conflicts which need to be tackled.

work through the night. They are most suitable for dry and older skins; those with oily, combination or normal skins may find that a daytime moisturiser is just as effective for night use. Night-time moisturisers are said to contain ingredients that 'feed' the skin as you sleep, but this is largely unproven.

Some creams are too heavy for delicate skin around the eyes and may cause irritation so special creams are used. Many eye creams are also claimed to reduce puffiness, minimise shadows and reduce fine lines.

Hands need regular applications of moisturiser as they are constantly exposed to air, frequent washing and contact with chemicals such as solvents. A layer of hand cream restores moisture and soothes the skin.

The skin on your body also needs moisturising because bathing and showering removes oils that need to be replaced. Regular exercisers tend to take more showers than others and so need extra skin care. Body lotions tend to be lighter and more easily absorbed than face creams, both for convenience and because the body skin is less exposed than the face and so does not require such a rich preparation.

Antiageing creams

Antiageing creams and lotions tighten the skin, minimising the appearance of fine lines, and rehydrate the top layer cells making the skin look smoother and more pliant.

Creams containing retinoic acid (a form of vitamin A) gradually remove layers of skin to reduce lines. Retinoic acid was used to treat acne for many years but scientific trials have now found that it can help reverse photoageing – the premature ageing of the skin caused by the sun. Retinoic acid can cause side effects such as skin flaking, dryness and reddening, and must be prescribed by a doctor.

AHAs (alpha-hydroxy acids), which occur naturally in fruit, vegetables and milk, are added to some moisturisers. They work by loosening the protein that glues the surface cells together, removing the outer layers of skin, accelerating cell renewal, and unblocking clogged pores. This makes the skin appear smoother and less lined. Sensitive skins may find that a high AHA level causes reddening and flaking. Choose a lower one – most products range from 1–10 per cent AHA. Stronger doses are available on prescription to treat acne.

SKIN TREATMENTS

The skin is constantly under assault from make-up, pollution, central heating, air conditioning and even hormonal changes. This can leave it looking tired, drawn, sallow and in need of a 'pick-me-up'. There is a range of beauty treatments on offer which aim to cleanse, moisturise and revitalise the skin. Although the health claims made for some treatments are unproven, there is evidence that regular beauty care keeps the skin clear, hydrated and blemish-free, and helps reduce fine lines.

Masks (or face packs) Applied to cleansed, moist skin these remove dead skin cells and other impurities, open the pores, and stimulate the circulation, making the skin smoother. The mask is left on for 10–15 minutes before removal. There are two types of mask: gel-like products that are washed off and mud masks which harden and must be peeled off. After removal of the mask, the skin should be rinsed with toner and, unless you have very oily skin, moisturiser should be applied.

Exfoliants (or scrubs) Containing gritty materials, these are massaged over the face to remove outer layers of epidermal cells and stimulate cell renewal to make the skin look and feel fresher and smoother. Some

NATURAL FACE SCRUB

This face scrub made from natural products not only removes dead skin cells and encourages the growth of new cells, it also feeds the skin, aids blood circulation and lymphatic drainage. Makes enough for two applications.

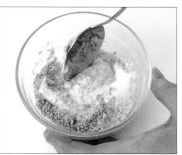

1 *In a bowl, mix 1 tbsp grapefruit juice, 2 tbsp medium oatmeal and ½ tbsp natural yoghurt until well combined into a paste.*

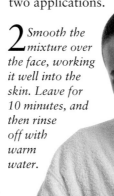

2 *Smooth the mixture over the face, working it well into the skin. Leave for 10 minutes, and then rinse off with warm water.*

THERAPEUTIC MUD BATHS

Mud baths work on the same principle as face packs but are applied to the whole body. Special types of mud, rich in vitamins, minerals and other trace elements, are said to have therapeutic properties as well as removing impurities from the skin. Therapeutic mud baths are very popular in continental Europe but there are mud spas to be found throughout the world. Depending on where the mud comes from, its active constituents vary. Therapeutic mud is used to treat conditions such as arthritis and rheumatism, skin disorders, reproductive disorders and digestive problems such as stomach ulcers. The most famous therapeutic mud is from Neydharting, Australia, and is exported worldwide for beauty treatments.

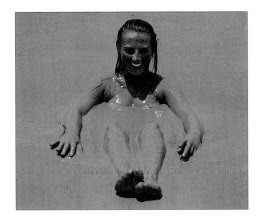

VOLCANIC SUPERMUD
Natural mud baths are found in countries with thermal or volcanic activity (often, the same country has both). Here, the volcanic mud naturally occurring in Arborettes in Colombia is thought to have healing powers.

exfoliants work by loosening the surface cells with chemicals, rather than by including abrasive substances.

Steaming This is a deep cleansing treatment that softens the skin, reduces oiliness, unblocks pores and removes blackheads. It is unsuitable for those prone to thread veins on the face as the heat dilates the blood vessels in the skin. To give yourself a steam treatment, pour boiling water into a bowl and add a few drops of essential oil suitable to your skin type (see page 62), stirring well. Lean over the bowl with a towel over your head and around the bowl to enclose your face with warm vapour. Keep in place for 5–10 minutes to allow the warm vapours to loosen dirt and grime and cleanse the pores.

A full facial Available at beauty salons, this combines various face treatments tailored to your skin type. First, make-up is removed and the skin thoroughly cleansed. The cleanser is removed with toner, and the face is steamed, with the eyes protected with moistened pads, containing a lotion to reduce puffiness. The next stage may be a moisturising mask or exfoliation, depending on skin type. Moisturising cream is then massaged into the face and neck, using sweeping upward movements.

A face massage As well as being relaxing, a face massage can help to reduce fine lines on the face and release tensed facial muscles, especially when used with lubricating oils or moisturisers. For a home massage, rub a little diluted essential oil on your fingertips and, starting on the inner eyebrows, make gentle, circular movements. Work your way up to the forehead, across to the temples, down to the cheekbones, across to the nose and down to the chin. Repeat, reversing the sequence.

Body massage Massage is beneficial for the whole body, especially when combined with aromatherapy, applying essential oils, which are absorbed through the pores and also inhaled. Aromatherapy massage can relieve stress, tension headaches, migraines, muscle strains, and menstrual and circulatory problems. Relaxing oils include frankincense, ylang ylang, neroli and myrrh. Stimulating oils include all of the citrus family as well as peppermint, pine and basil. For muscle strains try marjoram, cypress, hyssop, and black pepper. Oils for menstrual problems include geranium, camomile and jasmine. Circulatory problems can be eased with juniper, clary sage and ginger.

Body wrap This process involves covering the body with substances such as seaweed and algae and then wrapping it up in warmed towels to encourage the active constituents to be absorbed into the skin. It is claimed that the vitamins, minerals and enzymes in the plant material break down fat and water deposits, helping to detoxify the body and improve skin tone.

Turkish baths
Originating in the Middle East, Turkish baths have been established in the UK since the 19th century. The main feature of a Turkish bath is sitting or lying in a steam room filled with hot moist air where an all-over body massage takes place. To prepare the body for massage, you are asked to sit in a sauna then plunge into a cold water pool, alternating the two extremes a few times.

The humidity of the sauna and steam room removes toxins and excess fluid from the body's tissues and helps to alleviate conditions such as fluid retention, joint and muscle pain, and stress. People with circulatory or heart disorders should check with their doctor before having a Turkish bath.

FRUIT AND VEGETABLE SKIN BOOSTERS

The vitamins, minerals, enzymes and proteins in fruit and vegetables have a powerful action on the skin. Include at least five portions in your daily diet to give your skin extra protection. Antioxidants (vitamins C, E and beta carotene) work internally to neutralise harmful free radicals created by pollution and sunlight. Vitamin C is also required by the skin to make collagen, a form of protein which binds the skin and maintains its flexibility and strength. AHAs – natural acids found in many fruit and vegetables – stimulate the production of new skin cells. Examples of naturally occurring AHAs are mallic (found in apples) and pyruvic (found in papaya). Potassium is vital for controlling water balance in the body's tissues and cells.

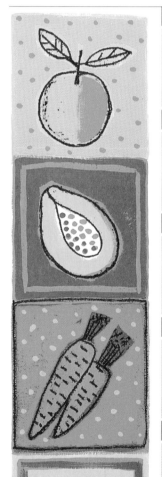

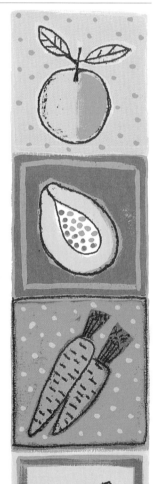

APPLE

Apple is high in pectin, which binds easily to toxic metals such as mercury and lead that may infiltrate the skin. It also has strong antiviral vitamin C, essential for skin healing.

AVOCADO

Rich in antioxidant vitamins A, C and E, and in potassium, avocado is also high in calories, so eat sparingly. Avocado is widely used in commercial skin preparations.

BEETROOT

Rich in iron, beetroot helps to purify the blood and remove toxins from the skin. It also has vitamins A and C for strong skin, and calcium for healthy nerves and bones.

CARROT

Carrot is a rich source of vitamins A, C and E, and beta carotene, as well as iron, calcium and potassium which help to form blood cells and promote strong bones.

GARLIC

Garlic has strong antiseptic, antibacterial, antiviral and antifungal properties. It is a natural detoxifier and antioxidant, and strengthens the immune system.

KELP AND SEAWEED

Kelp and seaweed are high in calcium, chromium, cobalt, iron, manganese, iodine and zinc which can help to clear the complexion. Ensure they are grown in pollutant-free water.

LIVE SPROUTS

Fresh live sprouts like alfalfa and bean sprouts are high in plant enzymes, essential fatty acids, B-complex vitamins and vitamins A, C and E. If left to grow nutrients will increase.

PARSLEY

Parsley is rich in beta carotene, vitamin C, calcium, iron, magnesium, phosphorus, potassium and chlorophyll and has traces of zinc and manganese.

CAPSICUM

Capsicums such as yellow and red peppers have very high levels of vitamin C. They are also high in beta carotene, iron and potassium – all good skin protectors.

WATERCRESS

Watercress is a powerful blood cleanser and helps to rid the body of toxins, making the skin clearer and healthier. It is also rich in A, C and E antioxidant vitamins.

PINEAPPLE

The inside of a pineapple makes an ideal exfoliant when rubbed over the skin. Pineapple is also good in facial treatments for problem skin. Eaten, it is a good source of vitamin C.

PAPAYA

An excellent source of vitamin C and beta carotene, papaya is also a good skincare product because it contains the fruit enzyme papain, which can be used to exfoliate and heal skin.

BANANA

Containing good levels of a wide range of vitamins and minerals including potassium and vitamin C, bananas are also used in many natural skincare products.

LEMON

Along with other citrus fruits, lemons are rich in vitamin C. In addition, the rind is packed with essential oils. Lemon juice can soften hard water and wash soap residues from skin.

Matching your style to your shape

Your personal style, shown in your choice of clothes and hairstyle, can play an important role in enhancing your shape and accentuating your best features.

Although diet and exercise can alter overall appearance, your essential shape – the structure of your bones and muscles and distribution of body fat – will be largely unchanged throughout your life. The way you dress can help you make the most of your natural assets and draw attention away from problem areas. Other factors, however, such as wearing high heels or carrying bags wrongly, can cause bad posture and misalignment in the body.

THE IMPORTANCE OF UNDERWEAR

What you wear underneath your clothes can make all the difference to your shape and overall appearance. Many large department stores offer a free fitting service with trained staff able to give advice and assistance on choosing the right underwear for you.

A properly fitting bra is one of the most important factors in influencing a woman's posture and appearance. The suspensory ligaments which support the breasts naturally stretch with time, allowing the breasts to sag. A bra lends support to these ligaments and helps keep the breasts firm and well-shaped. A bra is especially important during exercise when strenuous movement puts the suspensory ligaments under extra strain, with a greater risk of stretching. A strong, well-fitting sports bra avoids this problem by holding the breasts securely in place.

Ill-fitting bras can throw the body out of balance causing bad posture. If the back strap of the bra rides up, for example, it can put pressure on the shoulder blades and the base of the neck – a problem most often found in large-breasted women. The shoulders may also push back to compensate for a lack of support, or hunch over to hide a bra that accentuates a large bust.

Figure-shaping underwear

Support garments can improve your shape, pulling in your waist and flattening the stomach, but most have drawbacks. They can restrict the body's natural functions, such as breathing and digestion. The back muscles may come to rely on the support provided by corsets, for example, which can seriously weaken the spine. The abdominal muscles can lose tone through extended girdle wearing, leading to the build up of fat

THE ROLE OF THE SUSPENSORY LIGAMENTS

A woman's breasts are supported by strips of connective tissue called the suspensory ligaments of Cooper. These ligaments are connected to the muscles of the underarm, shoulders and chest. These muscles are a vital part of the breast support structure. Exercises that tone and strengthen them will also help to maintain firm breasts.

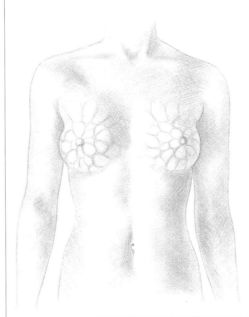

BREAST 'SLING'
The ligaments of Cooper form a sling-like arrangement that gives support to the breasts. However, the 'sling' is inelastic so that once it is stretched and the breasts drop, they cannot return to their former position. A bra gives vital extra support and should be worn from puberty when the breasts start to gain in size and weight. An extra-supportive bra is needed when the ligaments are put under increased strain, such as when playing sport or breastfeeding.

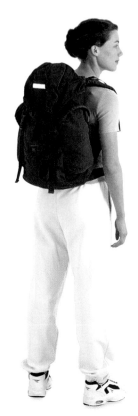

*DISTRIBUTING WEIGHT
EVENLY
Carrying heavy bags on
one shoulder can throw
your back out of
alignment, leading to
shoulder, back and neck
problems. To ensure that
any weight you carry is
distributed evenly, use a
backpack, correctly fitted
over both shoulders. If
you use a handbag or
work bag, choose one
with a shoulder strap and
carry the weight from the
opposite shoulder.*

and sagging. In addition, support garments do not solve the problem of excess fat but simply relocate it, often producing bulges in other areas of the body. It is much better to challenge weight problems with exercise and dietary measures before resorting to figure-shaping underwear, although, like high heels, occasional wear does little harm.

SHOES

No part of your outfit will dictate the way you look and feel as much as your footwear. During exercise, foot support is particularly important. There is a wide range of exercise footwear available and it is advisable to seek advice in selecting the right shoe for the activity you will be doing. A trainer intended for tennis, for example, will differ from one for aerobics. For day-to-day living, wear comfortable shoes that fit well but do not pinch. Women should avoid wearing high heels on a regular basis and instead aim for flat shoes or ones with a slightly raised heel, which allow ease of movement but offer a small lift to set off your clothes.

High heels and a woman's shape

In general, women like wearing high heels and men like the look of women wearing them. This is because they make the legs appear longer and the feet look smaller – both considered attractive characteristics. They also distort the posture, pushing the pelvis forward and forcing the lower back to arch and the bottom and the belly to stick out. The effect is sexually powerful, but the distortion to the spine and posture can negate any benefits. By wearing high heels, the body weight is balanced on the ball of the foot, which causes instability and weakening of the joints and muscles, especially in the ankle and the lower back. It also squeezes toes to the front of shoes, which causes bunions and other malformations.

ACCESSORIES

Accessories, particularly belts, can enhance and flatter your shape. Women often use items such as scarves and shawls, jewellery, hats, handbags, gloves and glasses to set off their outfits, but it is important that women do not allow accessories to overwhelm their appearance. In general, small accessories help to make a petite women appear in proportion. Larger accessories look better on large people.

Belts can be used to draw in the waist and emphasise the body's shape, but people who lack a waistline, having either a rounded or straight figure, should avoid drawing attention to the waist with a belt. Women with well-defined waistlines, especially those with larger hips and busts, benefit from wearing a narrow belt.

Shoulder pads in women's clothes and shoulder reinforcements in men's suits and jackets, give lift and balanced structure to your figure. They can also help to take the emphasis away from a thickening waistline or large stomach. Shoulder pads balance the shape of those with a fuller figure or a large bust but should be avoided by those with large or square shoulders as they will make you look top-heavy. Women should avoid wearing both a dress and a jacket with shoulder pads as this will overexaggerate the shoulders. Women can also use scarves and shawls to accentuate the shoulders, drawing attention away from large busts and stomachs.

Bags, handbags and backpacks

It is important to consider the effect on your posture of different bags and the way they are carried to avoid developing aches and pains in the back and shoulders. A single bag always unbalances the body by altering the centre of gravity, pulling one side down and putting the shoulders out of alignment.

Part of looking and feeling good is to be relaxed and unburdened. Learning how to carry bags properly can avoid pain and help you to feel relaxed and confident. According to experts, women carry far too much in their shoulder bags: 5.4 kg (12 lbs) is recommended as the maximum weight to carry on a regular basis, and ideally the weight should be distributed evenly over both shoulders in a backpack or satchel.

IMPROVING YOUR SHAPE WITH STYLE MANAGEMENT

Using clothes and style tricks to emphasise your best features and hide your worst can make all the difference to your appearance. Look at your body in a mirror and decide, as objectively as you can, which parts you want to emphasise and which parts you would rather conceal.

You can then work on different combinations of clothes to find the right balance for you. Different styles of clothes complement certain shapes and work against others. Men with a classic inverted triangle shape, for example, often appear top-heavy, especially if they wear long jackets or coats with reinforced shoulders. A softer look, removing the emphasis from the shoulders, can balance the shape. Tight-fitting tops and shirts which accentuate muscular shoulders and chest should be avoided. An open neckline breaks a wide shoulder-line, helping it to appear smaller, while tucking tops in at the waist helps to prevent a stocky appearance. Loose, pleated trousers will give the lower part of the body more bulk.

De-emphasising height

Tall people often feel that they appear overwhelming and may try to compensate by stooping, which is bad for the back. It is much better to balance your tall figure with well-chosen clothes. Wear jackets that cover your bottom (shorter jackets will exaggerate your height) but avoid long coats. Using several different colours or patterns in your outfit will break up your outline and help to reduce your apparent height. Tall women benefit from wearing loose-fitting trousers and fuller dresses. Short or knee-length skirts reduce leg length, especially when worn with a long, loose-fitting blouse or jumper. Men should wear properly fitting trousers, not too tight or too loose.

Disguising the stomach

The problem of how to disguise a large stomach is a common dilemma. Drawing attention to another part of the body is often one of the best strategies. Men should choose long jackets with reinforced shoulders which help to hide the abdomen and draw attention to the shoulders. Loose trousers help to balance the abdomen and legs, evening out your proportions. Loose shirts and tops, tucked into the trousers, will help to diminish stomach size.

Rounded women should aim to extend their overall length by drawing attention to the legs, face and neckline and away from

---

FLATTER YOUR BODY SHAPE

Although diet and exercise can help you to lose weight and tone your body, your basic shape will remain unchanged. This is where clothes can play a useful role in helping you to look in proportion. The right outfit will emphasise your best points as well as drawing attention away from problem areas.

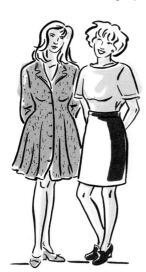

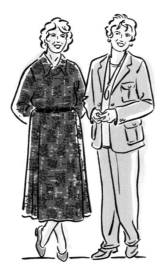

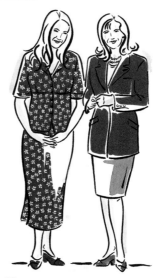

LARGE HIPS
Wear darker colours, plain colours or vertical stripes on your lower half. Pleats, bulky fabrics or outfits with a nipped-in waist will make your hips look bigger.

ROUNDED SHAPE
Choose clothes to elongate your figure. Wear tailored jackets with small shoulder pads. Avoid details such as belts, pleats or gathers which draw attention to the waist.

TALL WOMEN
To avoid looking taller than you are, avoid long-line skirts or dresses with small or fussy patterns. Opt for outfits in bold colours and wear more dramatic accessories.

Hair and your shape
Your hairstyle is an integral part of your personal style. Follow these simple guidelines for a style that complements the shape of your face:

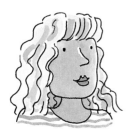

SQUARE FACE
Soften the lines of a square face by framing it with a fringe and curls or long waves at the sides.

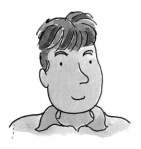

ROUND FACE
Choose a style that is shorter at the sides but is full at the crown to give more length to the face.

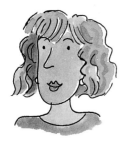

LONG FACE
A wavy style that is full at the sides, but short at the crown, helps to balance a long face.

the waist. V-necks, soft collars, scarves and necklaces complement the face and neckline. Long, loose-fitting jackets, blouses and jumpers, especially with padded shoulders, help to even out your proportions. Knee-length skirts and culottes draw attention to the legs, but shorts should be avoided.

Both sexes should choose plain patterns and muted colours. Avoid stripes and check patterns, which accentuate the outline.

Increasing stature
Tall, thin men can sometimes look shapeless and lacking in substance. Clothes that give shape can help to reduce this effect. It is important to ensure that your garments are not baggy, however, as this tends to give the impression of being too small for one's clothes. Reinforced shoulders can fill out the upper half of the body and draw attention to the shoulders. Properly fitting trousers help to make the body look in proportion. Baggy or pleated trousers should be avoided. Choose horizontal stripes which make the body appear broader and reduce the length. Avoid vertical stripes which have the opposite effect. V-necks and open shirt collars tend to elongate the face, making it look thinner; round-necked tops and jumpers are a better choice.

The most important rule for petite women is to wear small, well-fitted clothes with small prints or patterns. Wearing a single colour has the effect of elongating your outline, while multiple colours tend to break up your shape, making you look smaller.

Short jackets, especially waist-length, prevent you from appearing overwhelmed by your clothes. Knee-length or short, well-fitted skirts can make you appear less bulky. Well-fitted or figure-hugging trousers enhance your figure. Trousers that finish just above the ankle lengthen the legs. Baggy shirts and blouses can make you look dumpy; fitted tops and shirts are better.

Tips for women with large hips
Women with large hips can draw attention away from this area and accentuate the upper body instead. This can be achieved by using stronger colours and patterns on the top half and emphasising the shoulders. Wear long, loose-fitting jackets with wide lapels and loose tops to make the hips appear narrower. Padded shoulders, epaulettes, puffed sleeves, wide-necked tops,

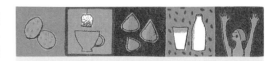

scarves and shawls will all help to make the shoulders and neckline appear wider and balance the hips. Choose skirts with pastel or pale floral designs contrasting with darker coloured or patterned tops.

Don't wear pleated dresses and skirts that are too tight over the hips making them look even bigger than they are. Pattern details, motifs and pockets on the hips should also be avoided.

Tips for women with large busts
Large-busted women should aim to draw attention away from the upper body. Lowering the waistline makes the bust seem more in proportion with the rest of the body. You can broaden and lengthen the appearance of the upper body by wearing long, loose-fitting jackets, tops and jumpers, especially with wide shoulders, shoulder pads, and V-necklines. It is best to avoid short sleeves, collars and high necklines.

Wear long dresses with belts worn low on the hips and avoid high-waisted skirts. Avoid short tops and jackets, especially with breast pockets, stripes or fussy detail around the lapels.

C H A P T E R 4

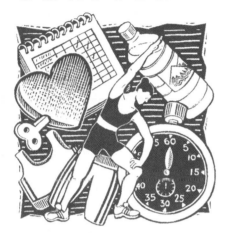

YOUR SHAPING-UP PROGRAMME

A shaping-up programme needs to be carefully planned. Setting your exercise goals and knowing which exercises burn fat and which build muscle strength will help you to tailor your regime to your individual requirements. Understanding how the muscles work and how best to improve their strength and flexibility will help you to target specific areas to improve your shape and posture.

SETTING YOUR SHAPING-UP GOALS

The starting point for any exerciser is to determine what you want to achieve from your shaping-up programme, be it weight reduction, body toning, or building muscle strength.

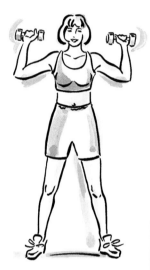

***WHAT IS PROGRESSIVE RESISTANCE EXERCISE?** Progressive resistance training is defined as any muscular work that is performed against a resistance, such as a weight, with the aim of increasing muscular strength and tone. Typically, this resistance takes the form of free weights such as barbells and dumbbells or fixed weights such as those found in gyms.*

A shaping-up programme needs to be tailored to your goals. It is surprising, therefore, that many people set out on an exercise regime with no clear idea of what they want it to achieve.

DECIDING ON YOUR GOALS

Before designing an exercise programme it is important to know what you are aiming to achieve. The human body has the capacity to transform itself in many different ways, responding to how it is challenged. Regular stretching of the muscles, for example, can result in greater range of movement, while resistance training leads to increased muscular tone.

To decide if you are overweight for your height, work out your BMI (see page 16). It will be particularly important to combine exercise with a controlled diet, low in fat and high in complex carbohydrates, to achieve and maintain weight-loss goals. You may also need to focus on aerobic forms of exercise such as brisk walking, swimming or cycling, as forms of exercise that demand greater use of oxygen are more efficient at burning fat (see page 83).

Aerobic exercise should also be the focus of your programme if you want to improve your general level of fitness. Aerobic exercise improves the functioning of your heart and lungs, the foundations of good general health. As your muscles are worked they in turn demand extra oxygen from your body. The heart pumps more oxygen-carrying blood around your body, improving its strength and efficiency over time.

If your weight and general fitness level is good, you can begin to focus your shaping-up programme on muscle toning and strength building. If you want to improve the bulk of your muscles you will need to perform high-resistance exercises, for example, lifting heavier weights over shorter periods of time. However, if you simply want to firm your muscles up without necessarily increasing bulk, you will need to perform muscular endurance work. In these kinds of exercises, resistance (the weight you are working against) is only moderate, and the emphasis is on working over longer periods.

Whatever your overall goals, in order for the body to move freely joints need to maintain good ranges of movement. You can

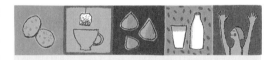

SUPER SHAPER

Swimming is a low-impact exercise which doesn't put strain on the body, as it is supported by the buoyancy of the water. With each stroke, muscles are lengthened and strengthened – water is 12 times as resistant as air. Continuous swimming provides a good aerobic work-out for the heart and lungs and can boost energy levels. Aqua aerobics (aerobics in water) is a good alternative for people who don't enjoy swimming lengths. It can be easier than normal aerobics classes yet gives the same effect because of the resistance of the water. There are also water exercise classes specially designed for pregnant women. Because the buoyancy of the water eliminates stress on joints, it is a safe way to exercise and tone the body even late into a pregnancy.

DID YOU KNOW?

During exercise your heart rate speeds up to pump a greater volume of blood to the muscle groups being used. Depending on the type and intensity of the exercise, the amount of blood pumped around the body can increase from the usual 4 litres a minute to 27 litres (9 to 54 pints).

achieve this through daily stretching of surrounding muscles. Healthy and flattering posture is not only dependent on sufficient muscular tone but also good flexibility. Your shape can improve dramatically simply as a result of holding yourself in better alignment and maintaining poised posture.

Finally, when setting goals try to make sure they are realistic and attainable. Some people are born with body types best adapted for endurance. The narrow shoulders and hips of long-distance runners, along with their naturally lean body composition, can never be transformed into the heavier, broad shape seen among power lifters.

The secret to success is making the most of what you have. Attempts to transform your body into something it is not meant to be are ultimately self-defeating.

CONSULT YOUR GP

Before starting your new exercise routine it is a good idea to have a medical check-up, especially if you are older or unaccustomed to vigorous activity.

Remember that most GPs have no more knowledge of what various exercise programmes involve than the average person, so it is helpful for you to give them a brief, yet clear, outline of what you intend to do and achieve. If you have sought advice from a fitness professional (see right) then they will be able to compile a written description of the proposed activity which you can then take along to show your doctor.

Medical check-ups primarily focus on identifying any existing risk factors for cardiovascular disease. You can expect to be asked questions regarding the health status of your biological parents and grandparents, your dietary habits, tobacco use, alcohol consumption and stress levels. Your blood pressure will be taken and your heart listened to for any irregularities. It is possible that your cholesterol levels will also be tested. Be sure to discuss any other issues with your doctor that may affect the level to which you are able to exercise safely, such as arthritis, back problems, recent or old injuries and joint or muscular concerns.

Getting advice

The better informed you become prior to undertaking a new exercise programme, the safer and more effective it is likely to be. Seek advice from professionals such as properly qualified fitness experts. Employing the services of a personal trainer, at least in the initial stages of a new regime, is strongly recommended. Your local leisure centre should be able to put you in contact with a qualified trainer. Additionally, refer to the many fitness books and publications available at your local library.

WORKING EFFECTIVELY WITHIN SAFE LIMITS

Like other muscles, your heart can be trained to increase performance, but there are limits to what can be termed as safe training. To stick within these limits, it is useful to work out your target training zone. Take your pulse 30 seconds after energetic exercise to check if you are working safely within your target zone. Over time, increase the intensity of your training but never work to your maximum heart rate (maximum heart rate = 220 minus your age).

TAKING YOUR PULSE DURING TRAINING
Using two fingers, find your pulse at the inside of your wrist near your thumb. As your pulse will be slowing down, count the beats for 15 seconds, then multiply this count by four.

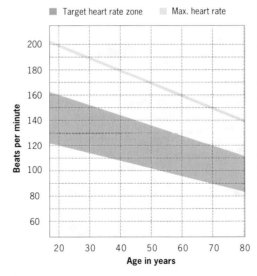

FINDING YOUR TRAINING ZONE
This graph shows average target heart rate and maximum heart rates according to age. You should aim to exercise at between 65 and 85 per cent of your maximum.

Best of both worlds

By combining resistance training and regular aerobic activity you will improve your body shape as well as your overall fitness level. Aerobic exercise increases the efficiency of the heart, lungs and circulatory system, while resistance work increases muscle strength and tone.

MONITORING YOUR PROGRESS

The establishment of long-term goals can be a powerful motivational tool, but breaking them down into a series of progressive stages is less daunting, and provides attainable short-term aims. Be realistic regarding the time span you allow for your achievements and be prepared to adapt your plan as necessary. Both long and short-term goals need to be specific and measurable.

With regard to body weight remember that the bathroom scales offer little insight into your fat/muscle ratio. Scales only show you your overall total body weight which, due to fluid fluctuations, can vary even from day to day. A better way to monitor your progress is to mix the factors being measured. It can be very encouraging to measure improvements in your pulse rate taken at rest as this will indicate a rise in your basic level of fitness. Keeping a note of your waist and hip measurements can be helpful; in addition simply keeping a diary in which you record your responses to your training regime may provide an interesting record, hopefully revealing improvements in the amount of exercise you can perform and the ease with which you can perform it.

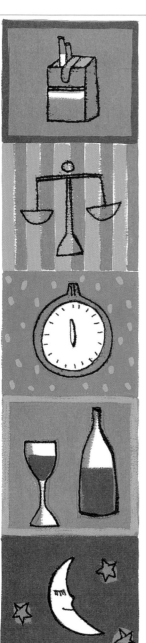

HOW MUCH DO YOU NEED TO SHAPE UP?

The aim and course of your shaping-up programme will be determined by your health and level of fitness at the outset.

This quiz will help you to decide how much you need to shape up and on which areas your programme should focus.

Do you get very breathless as a response to:	When buying clothes do you find getting a good fit:	Do you suffer from aches and pains:
(a) walking up stairs (b) walking briskly (c) jogging (d) exercising hard?	(a) very difficult (b) often a problem (c) sometimes a problem (d) no problem?	(a) constantly (b) often (c) occasionally (d) rarely?
Do you smoke:	Are your energy levels:	Do you have difficulty in sleeping:
(a) frequently (b) socially (c) seldom (d) never?	(a) generally low (b) they fluctuate quite a lot (c) okay most of the time (d) generally high?	(a) a lot of the time (b) sometimes (c) once in a while (d) rarely?
Is your BMI:	Do you suffer from low spirits:	Do you suffer from stiff joints:
(a) obese (b) overweight (c) on the margin of overweight (d) appropriate to your height?	(a) frequently (b) occasionally (c) sometimes, but it's manageable (d) seldom?	(a) constantly (b) frequently after exercise (c) sometimes after intense exercise (d) seldom?
Do you drink alcohol to excess:	Do you take exercise:	Is your resting heart rate:
(a) every day (b) once a week (c) once a month (d) rarely?	(a) seldom (b) occasionally (c) once or twice a week (d) more than twice a week?	(a) poor (b) fair (c) good (d) excellent?

Mostly 'a's: First, you need to improve your general level of health with the guidance of your doctor. Your shaping-up programme should focus on aerobic exercise to improve your cardiovascular health, but you should also look at other lifestyle factors such as diet.

Mostly 'b's: Your general level of fitness could be improved with aerobic exercise. This will help you to control weight problems, and may help to overcome any joint stiffness or low energy levels.

Mostly 'c's: Your general level of fitness is probably quite reasonable but there will still be areas in which you can improve. Your shaping-up programme can focus more on toning your body and increasing your flexibility and strength to achieve a shape you're happy with.

Mostly 'd's: Your general level of fitness is very good. However, it is easy to let fitness slip. Your programme should focus on muscle toning and maintaining your current activity levels.

THE IMPORTANCE OF STRETCHING

Whatever form of exercise you choose to undertake, proper stretching should be an integral part of your shaping-up programme, both before and after exercise.

Healthy shape is not only dependent on good muscle tone; in order to hold good body alignment and posture, as well as to control movement, flexibility is essential, and for good flexibility you need to stretch your muscles regularly. Stretching is also essential in helping to avoid strain, and can prevent injury.

HOW MUSCLES STRETCH

Our skeletal muscles are generally attached to bones via tendons at each end of the muscle. When contracting, a muscle shortens and exerts a pulling force on the bones. As the two ends of the muscle draw towards each other the bones move. In order to do this the muscle must cross a joint.

Muscles can only pull, they cannot push, and for this reason they always work in pairs with their partner crossing the opposite side of the joint. For example, it is the biceps that pull to flex the elbow but the triceps on the opposing side that pull to extend it (see page 80).

The range of movement around joints is therefore dependent not only on a muscle's ability to pull and create movement but also on its capacity to stretch and accommodate it. Flexibility training focuses on taking the two ends of any given muscle away from each other to challenge its ability to stretch.

HOW STRETCHING IMPROVES YOUR SHAPE

Posture describes the way in which bones are held up and carried by the skeletal muscles. When joints are correctly aligned, the nervous system and internal organs can function at optimal efficiency. Poor posture results in wasted energy and impedes the circulatory flow; the respiratory function decreases and digestive problems may occur. Regular use of misaligned joints can also lead to arthritis and chronic soft tissue injuries, as well as lower back pain.

You can transform your shape and appearance simply by improving your posture. A body carrying a few excess pounds of fat, but held with poise and grace, is a great improvement on a slender person who slouches; the person projects an image of self-confidence that is innately attractive.

DEVELOPMENTAL STRETCHING

Muscles have an in-built memory and automatically contract at their habitual limit. However, by holding a stretch until the muscle relaxes into the position, the limit can be taken further. This new flexibility is then logged in the muscle's memory, increasing the muscle's capability. The exercise below stretches the muscles of the inner thigh.

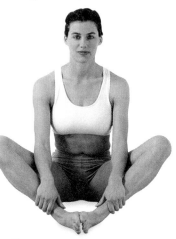

FIRST STAGE STRETCHING
Slowly ease your knees towards the floor. Hold for at least 10 seconds until you feel your muscles relax into the stretch.

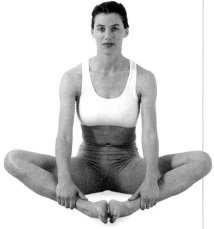

INCREASING THE STRETCH
Take the stretch further very slowly until you feel your muscles tensing once more. Hold for a minimum of 10 seconds.

The ability to achieve and maintain good posture depends on having both sufficient muscular tone and adequate flexibility. For example, the muscles of the upper back stop the shoulders collapsing forwards, but unless the chest can stretch to accommodate the position it will cause rounded shoulders.

When flexed positions are consistently adopted, the muscles around the joints can become shortened and inflexible. This is known as adaptive shortening and is often seen in people who spend much of their daily lives sitting. When you are seated, both the hips and knees are flexed, resulting in the hamstring muscles at the back of the thighs and the hip flexors at the front of the hip being in a shortened position. High-heeled shoes have a similar effect on calf muscles. The heel is unnaturally raised, resulting in bunching up of the muscles and their consequent loss of ability to extend.

Daily stretches for the muscles at the front of the chest, the backs of the thighs and, especially for women, the calf muscles will help the body to become sufficiently elastic to accommodate a better posture.

THE STRETCH REFLEX

To avoid the danger of being overextended, muscles have a self-protection mechanism which must be taken into account if stretching is to be safe and effective.

Every time the two ends of the muscle are taken to the limits of their range a warning signal is transmitted to the brain via sensory nerves (see page 91). In response, the brain commands the muscle to contract to protect itself. This means that whenever you stretch the initial result is actually a contraction. Only after the position has been held still and taken no further will the muscle relax. The time it takes for this reflex action to occur and then release is at least 6 seconds. Any stretch held for less than this amount of time is therefore ineffective.

METHODS OF STRETCHING

The most effective way to increase muscle elasticity is to perform what is known as developmental stretching, also known as proprioceptive muscular facilitation (PMF). The muscle is taken to the limits of its range where it is held statically for 10 seconds,

THE MECHANICS OF MUSCLE CONTRACTION

Skeletal muscles work in pairs to allow movement at a joint. As one muscle (the agonist) contracts, its opposite (the antagonist) must relax to allow the movement. If the antagonist is too short, for example, because of excessive tension or lack of exercise, movement will be restricted. A muscle that is too short will also impact on its opposite muscle, which can then become weak or overly stretched.

A muscle contains hundreds of elongated cells called muscle fibres (see page 87). Each fibre contains hundreds of myofibrils and it is the shortening that occurs within these that causes the muscle itself to contract.

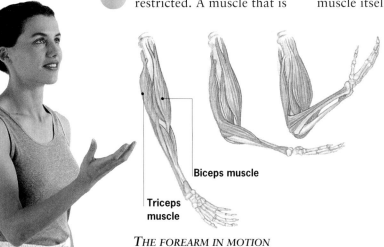

Biceps muscle

Triceps muscle

THE FOREARM IN MOTION
To raise the forearm, the biceps bulks up and its opposite muscle, the triceps, stretches to allow movement. To lower the arm, the triceps contracts and the biceps relaxes.

THE SHORTENING OF THE MYOFIBRIL
In contraction, the thick filaments contained in the myofibril slide in between the thin ones. It is this action which causes the muscle as a whole to contract.

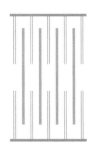

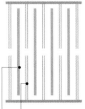

Thin filaments of actin
Thick filaments of myosin

In relaxed muscle
thick and thin filaments overlap slightly

In contracted muscle, the thick filaments slide in between the thin ones

or until you can feel the tension release. Once the stretch reflex has dispersed, and the muscle has relaxed, it may be eased further. Initially it will contract again and must be given time to relax into its new position. You can repeat this gentle progressive lengthening two or three times. It is most effective in improving range of movement if performed daily.

Take care not to bounce or 'pulse' when stretching as this continually triggers the stretch reflex and consequently leads to a build-up of tension within the muscle rather than the lengthening and relaxing needed to increase flexibility safely.

The more support the body has when stretching the more relaxed it will be; therefore performing stretches on the floor, where appropriate, is particularly useful.

EFFECTIVE STRETCHING

When one muscle's partner, on the other side of the joint, has to contract to bring about a stretch it is known as an active stretch. For example, from standing, the heel of one leg can be pulled up towards the bottom using the hamstrings on the back of the thigh. However, with so much tension in the back of the leg it is very difficult for the quadriceps, those that run down the front of the thigh, to relax into the stretch. A more effective stretch would be to use the muscles of the arm to hold the leg in position. In this way the entire thigh can relax. This method is known as passive stretching.

WHEN TO STRETCH

It is essential to lengthen your muscles prior to exercising, in order to maximise the range of movement. Gentle stretching of the major muscle groups such as the hamstrings at the back of the thigh and the adductors on the inner thigh, may also reduce the likelihood of injury. Pre-exercise stretches need to be held for a minimum of 10 seconds to be effective. Focus particularly on those muscles that will be involved in the activity you are about to do.

For developmental stretching to be safe and effective, muscles need to increase in pliability, and to do this they must produce heat via movement. Attempting to stretch cold muscles may result in damage. Brisk walking, gentle cycling or even vigorous housework can all raise muscle temperature and enhance elasticity. Stretching is most efficient when the muscles are at their warmest, that is after vigorous activity.

Stretching after exercise has shown to be helpful in reducing muscle soreness sometimes felt 24–48 hours after a tough workout. The relaxed lengthening of muscles, and consequent reduction in their tension, also has a calming effect on the mind and can help to ensure a sound night's sleep.

Before designing your stretch programme, identify where you feel adequately flexible and which joints feel restricted in their ranges of movement. Where muscles are already flexible, performing regular static stretches of 8–10 seconds duration will maintain their elasticity. For those muscles that are tight, and limited in their range, try performing daily developmental stretches.

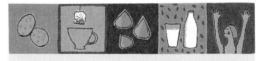

SUPER SHAPER

Jogging is an excellent way to warm up before a stretching session and thanks to mini trampolines (or trampets), you don't even have to leave the house. This inexpensive item of home equipment provides ideal aerobic activity. It's up to you how you use it – you could simply jog normally or you could bounce, lifting your arms above your head and down again as you do so. Make sure the legs of the trampet are secure and there is enough head room for safe exercising. If you are a keen jogger, a trampet means you are not limited to jogging in daylight hours and need not go out when the weather is bad.

BALLISTIC STRETCHING

Ballistic stretching uses fast, jerky or 'bounce' movements to increase a stretch. An example of this is bouncing to touch your toes. Ballistic stretches might be used by professional gymnasts prior to specific actions, but are generally not recommended for a number of reasons:

▶ *A rushed stretch does not allow enough time for tissues to adapt, resulting in strain.*

▶ *A sudden jerk to a muscle will initiate the stretch reflex and muscle tension will increase. Pulling against this tension can result in microscopic tears of the myofibrils. Healing will result in the formation of fibrous tissue which impairs muscle function.*

▶ *Bouncing movements are not easy to control. Therefore the positioning of joints and the direction of movement may not be correct, increasing the likelihood of injury.*

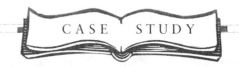
A Headache Sufferer

The healthy functioning of your body is greatly affected by the way you hold yourself. Today's sedentary lifestyle can result in muscles that are too weak and inflexible for good posture. Poor diet and high stress levels compound the problem. By increasing muscle tone and flexibility through exercise, your body shape, health and energy levels can all be improved.

Rita is a 31-year-old computer programmer who recently returned to part-time work following the birth of her second child. She has suffered digestive problems since college and during her pregnancy was diagnosed with irritable bowel syndrome (IBS), but since returning to work she has started to feel run-down. She gets frequent headaches and has a stubborn respiratory infection, which she blames for her general aches and pains. She knows her diet could be better – neither she nor her husband Peter are great cooks, and they eat a lot of ready-prepared foods. She also feels she needs more exercise, but with young children it is not easy to find the time.

WHAT SHOULD RITA DO?

The rushed, unhealthy diet and day-to-day stress are not helping Rita's health, but many of her problems stem from poor posture at work. She needs a better diet – balanced, nutritious meals do not have to involve great amounts of cooking time or skill – and daily periods of exercise and relaxation. At work, she must ensure that her computer is positioned to allow her to sit upright without tilting forwards. Muscular toning and stretching will improve her health and posture. Simple, corrective exercises for 2-3 minutes every hour can strengthen the upper back muscles, realign the cervical vertebrae and expand the chest, so aiding the digestive system.

Action Plan

EMOTIONAL HEALTH
Find some time each day for relaxation – especially at the end of the day to promote sound sleep.

DIET
Eat plenty of fresh fruit and vegetables every day – raw, where possible. Start keeping a food diary to try to identify if certain foods spark off the IBS.

LIFESTYLE
Spend some time each day outdoors. Include some exercise each day, even if it's just taking the children to the park.

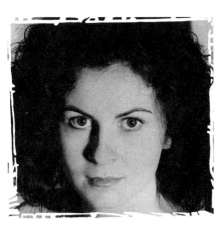

LIFESTYLE
Fresh air, natural light and exercise are vital for both health and emotional well-being.

EMOTIONAL HEALTH
It is easy to forget your own needs when a family is making demands on your time and energy.

DIET
Processed foods can cause digestive distress. Caffeine and condiments are intestinal irritants. Simple wholesome meals are the best choice.

HOW THINGS TURNED OUT FOR RITA

Rita had her computer raised to prevent her slouching and is now aware of her posture so does some stretches every hour. At home, she makes an effort to get out with the children every day and at weekends the whole family goes for a walk. She and Peter are both learning to cook, and now feel their diet is much better. Rita has fewer headaches, the IBS is much improved, and she has far more energy than before.

THE PHYSIOLOGY OF FAT BURNING

If the main aim of your shaping-up programme is to lose weight, it will undoubtedly help you to have an understanding of how fat is formed, stored and utilised in the body.

The term 'fat' is used to describe a collection of thin-walled, oil-filled cells that mostly lie just beneath the skin. Each pound of fat stored in the body is the equivalent of 3000–3500 calories.

Fat is essential in our diet, helping to make available valuable fat-soluble A, D, E and K vitamins, promoting healthy skin and for regulating body functions. However, most dietitians agree that the average Western person eats more fat than is required or is good for health. Excess fat that cannot be utilised as a fuel source by your body is stored as fat cells within the skin. Over time this can lead to problems with weight, and to cardiovascular disorders. Most people understand that exercise can help to utilise excess fat stores in the body, but how exactly does this occur?

HOW EXERCISE BURNS FAT

For muscles to contract they must have a continual supply of phosphates, which the body provides by breaking down food. Carbohydrates are required in the greatest quantities, as it is from these that phosphates are most readily obtained. When consumed, carbohydrates are converted into either glycogen, glucose, or fat. Glycogen is stored primarily in the liver and muscles where it is available to provide phosphates

continued on page 86

BURNING FAT THROUGH DIET AND EXERCISE

In order to burn fat, exercise and diet must be considered. Studies show that the best way to burn fat is by performing low-intensity aerobic exercise for at least 20 minutes three times a week. Fat can only be converted to energy by the presence of oxygen. Short, intense bursts of activity such as a quick sprint are anaerobic exercise, which means they do not use oxygen and utilise energy sources in the body other than fat. An hour's brisk walk, however, gets your cardiovascular system pumping oxygen to your muscles and mobilises fat stores. Combined with a low-fat diet, this is the best way to burn fat.

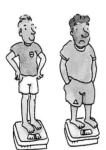

A healthy weight means you are eating the right amount of food for your activity levels. Overweight people eat more than they expend and so have excess stores of fat.

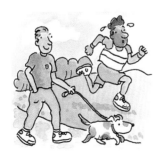

Regular, low-intensity exercise such as walking or cycling for an hour will burn fat more effectively than short, intense bursts of exercise.

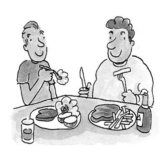

Following a low-fat diet will provide the right form of fuel for increased activity. High-fat food is less readily converted to energy by your body and so is stored as fat.

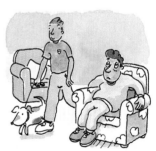

Your energy levels will be high as your body easily converts complex carbohydrates to fuel. With a high-fat diet you are more likely to feel fatigued by increased activity.

Starting Exercise for the

Very Overweight

The less fit you are the harder exercising becomes. For those carrying a lot of excess weight, the challenge can seem daunting. But by planning a programme that is easy to perform, exercise can quickly become enjoyable – and show results.

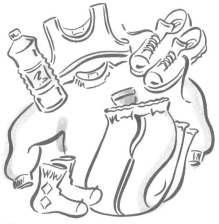

EQUIPPED FOR ACTION
Wear loose, comfortable clothing made of natural fibres that allow your body to breathe and will absorb moisture. Dress in layers so that clothes can be removed as you warm up. The ideal footwear is a pair of aerobic trainers. Always have a bottle of water to hand to make sure you don't get dehydrated.

Many heavily overweight individuals feel embarrassed to exercise in public and so try to lose weight by diet alone. This method is unlikely to achieve the desired result; it often leads to yo-yo dieting and, consequently, a slower metabolic rate, which compounds the weight problem. Whatever your weight, the combination of a low-fat diet and well-planned, regular aerobic exercise is the quickest route to successful slimming and an increased feeling of well-being. Exercise will also boost your metabolism and firm up flabby areas so that your clothes will fit better even before you actually lose weight. Before you start to exercise be sure you are dressed comfortably – for large-breasted women, a well-supporting bra is essential.

Excess body weight puts an unnatural pressure on the joints, so to protect the weight-bearing joints when exercising be sure to begin with flexibility exercises.

Always perform the movements slowly, aiming to achieve the biggest possible range of motion.

FLEXIBILITY EXERCISES

Most people reach peak flexibility around the age of ten. As you age, your range of movement gradually reduces and as muscles and tendons around joints shorten, stiffness can occur. This process often takes place quicker in overweight people as they find themselves doing less and less exercise and their muscles become conditioned to a limited range of movement. The most common areas affected are the knees, lower back, hips, fingers and toes. With regular stretching, however, which takes your muscles beyond their normal range, you can slowly increase your flexibility and enjoy greater ease of movement.

ANKLE FLEXOR
Sitting in a chair, point and flex each foot ten times, then circle the ankles ten times in each direction.

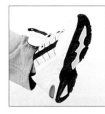
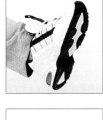
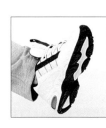

CIRCLING
Circle each foot with a slow and controlled movement.

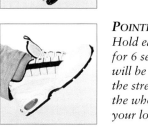

POINTING
Hold each point for 6 seconds. You will be able to feel the stretch along the whole length of your lower leg.

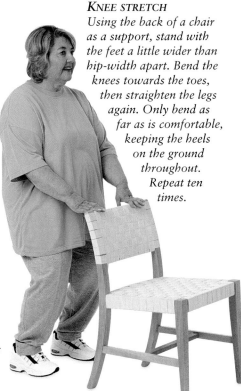

KNEE STRETCH
Using the back of a chair as a support, stand with the feet a little wider than hip-width apart. Bend the knees towards the toes, then straighten the legs again. Only bend as far as is comfortable, keeping the heels on the ground throughout. Repeat ten times.

AEROBIC EXERCISES

A common problem for heavily overweight people during exercise is skin burn. This occurs when one part of the body rubs against another when moving, resulting in chafing. Skin burn most commonly occurs on the inner thighs and underarms. The following exercises avoid this while being effective aerobic conditioners. The number of times you repeat an aerobic exercise before moving on to the next can be increased as your fitness improves. Begin with ten repetitions of each exercise and work up to 20. Once you can perform each exercise 20 times comfortably, aim to do the entire routine a second time. You may need to reduce the repetitions in the second run through to ten until your stamina improves. A good aim is eventually to be able to repeat the whole sequence six times through, performing each exercise 20 times.

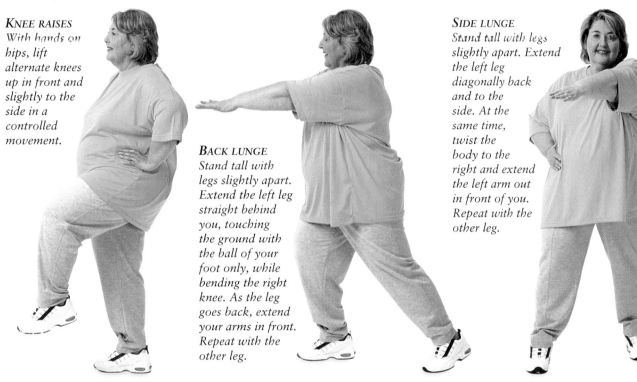

KNEE RAISES
With hands on hips, lift alternate knees up in front and slightly to the side in a controlled movement.

BACK LUNGE
Stand tall with legs slightly apart. Extend the left leg straight behind you, touching the ground with the ball of your foot only, while bending the right knee. As the leg goes back, extend your arms in front. Repeat with the other leg.

SIDE LUNGE
Stand tall with legs slightly apart. Extend the left leg diagonally back and to the side. At the same time, twist the body to the right and extend the left arm out in front of you. Repeat with the other leg.

WARMING UP AND COOLING DOWN

Start by performing some basic stretches for the back, legs and shoulders (see Chapter 5). To allow your body to adapt gradually to the demands of the exercises, go through them slowly first without the arm work, then introduce the arms and up the tempo as you feel more confident. Suddenly stopping after continuous activity can cause dizziness and contribute to the formation of varicose veins. To prevent this, finish each session by repeating the movements slowly, keeping the hands on the hips.

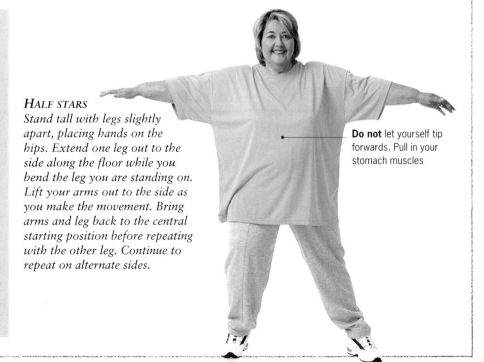

HALF STARS
Stand tall with legs slightly apart, placing hands on the hips. Extend one leg out to the side along the floor while you bend the leg you are standing on. Lift your arms out to the side as you make the movement. Bring arms and leg back to the central starting position before repeating with the other leg. Continue to repeat on alternate sides.

Do not let yourself tip forwards. Pull in your stomach muscles

for muscle contraction. Glucose circulates in the blood to feed the brain, kidneys and red blood cells. Once glycogen and glucose stores are replenished, any extra carbohydrates are stored as fat, mostly under the skin and around the internal organs.

Although proteins are also a potential source of phosphates, their main role is to provide materials for cell building. Once the body's protein needs are met, any excess will be converted to fat for storage.

Fat is a potential source of fuel, but in order for fat to be broken down for fuel, oxygen must be present. This means that most of the fat that we eat is transferred directly into the fat stores of the body.

Many people believe that the intensity at which you perform exercise is the key to burning fat, but this is not necessarily the case. Aerobic exercise, which utilises oxygen as the energy source, is the most effective at burning fat, and the longer it is performed the more fat will be utilised. If the intensity of the exercise causes you to become out of breath, this is a sign that the oxygen supply is insufficient and therefore fat cannot be utilised. Forms of exercise such as weightlifting, sprinting or ballet, which involve sudden bursts of extreme activity, do not use the aerobic system. They use the anaerobic (without oxygen) systems, which provide instant but unsustainable energy gained from glycogen rather than fat. Lactic acid may be produced as a by-product, and as levels build up this is felt as a burning sensation in the muscles when exercising at high intensities.

THE TALK TEST
Exercise increases your heart rate, making you breathe harder, but being out of breath is a sign that you are overdoing it. It also means oxygen cannot be delivered to the muscle in time for fat burning so your body is predominantly breaking down glycogen for fuel instead of fat. When exercising with a friend, monitor your breathing by trying to hold a conversation. If you are exercising alone attempt to sing or recite a rhyme.

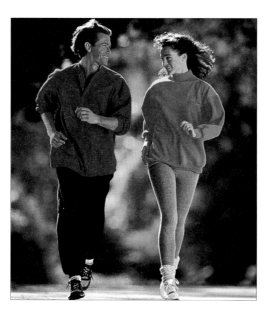

CHECK LIST
There are several ways of monitoring your progress during training:

✔ *Try the talk test (see below).*

✔ *Calculate your target training zone (see page 77) and check your pulse during training to make sure you stay within it.*

✔ *Take your resting pulse twice a week and keep a note of the count. A slower resting pulse indicates a fitness improvement.*

✔ *Use a scale of perceived exertion evaluated from 1 to 10, with 1 representing total inactivity and 10 maximum exertion. Effective fat burning for those unaccustomed to exercise takes place around 6 or 7 on the scale.*

✔ *Buy a heart rate monitor which straps around the chest and transmits the speed of cardiac contractions to a display worn on the wrist. An alarm will sound if you drop below or exceed your preset target heart rate.*

SPEEDING UP YOUR METABOLISM
While lower intensity, sustained exercise is the best way to utilise fat, higher intensity exercise is more effective at raising your metabolic rate. This is the rate at which your body utilises energy for all its basic functions. Exercise speeds up the resting metabolic rate (RMR) for some hours after exertion, meaning that more calories are burned up even when at rest.

The greater the intensity of exercise the faster the metabolism speeds up and the longer it remains elevated. Research shows that it can stay quicker for 24 hours or more after 30 minutes of vigorous activity.

Experts recommend at least 20 minutes of sustained aerobic exercise at least three times a week in order to achieve and maintain a moderate level of fitness. Obviously, the more exercise you do, the greater the fat-burning potential, but all experts agree that a little and often is much better than sporadic, intense bursts. The aim should be to make aerobic exercise a regular feature of your daily life.

THE PHYSIOLOGY OF MUSCLE BUILDING

Understanding how muscles work can help you to plan an effective exercise programme which will build up or strengthen muscles, and avoid damage through excess or incorrect use.

The muscles of your body have four characteristics that set them apart from other types of tissue. These are: excitability, the capacity to receive and respond to a nerve impulse; contractability, the ability to contract; extensibility, the ability to stretch; and elasticity, the capacity to return to their original shape. Any form of regular exercise which uses the muscles will therefore result in measurable changes in their tone and shape.

TYPES OF MUSCLE

There are three main types of muscle found in the body: heart, or cardiac, muscle, which has the capacity to beat at a constant steady rhythm without tiring; involuntary muscle, found, for example, in the gastrointestinal tract, which carries out other automatic functions; and voluntary or skeletal muscle, which is responsible for all conscious movement. It is the skeletal muscles, along with the skeleton and any stored fat, that determine your body shape.

Contractions by the skeletal muscles are designed to bring about movement or maintain posture. For example, when you are walking along carrying a heavy load, the leg muscles provide mobility while the arm muscles support the load and the muscles of the torso keep you upright. Skeletal muscles also produce a lot of heat energy – as much as 85 per cent of body heat – which is why exercise warms you up.

THE ANATOMY OF SKELETAL MUSCLE

It is the anatomy of skeletal muscles which enables them to contract. The muscle consists of dense groups of elongated cells called muscle fibres. These can be up to 30 cm (1 ft) long and are held together, in groups called fascicles, by a sheath of connective tissue called the perimysium. The muscle fibres are fed with oxygen and glucose by the many capillaries that break through the perimysium. Within each muscle fibre are bundles of thinner fibres

continued on page 90

INSIDE SKELETAL MUSCLE

Only one type of muscle, skeletal muscle, requires conscious direction from the brain to work. Nerves travel through the muscle carrying messages from the brain. To fulfil the demands made of them, skeletal muscles vary greatly in size, but they all have a similar construction which allows them to contract when stimulated by nerve impulses.

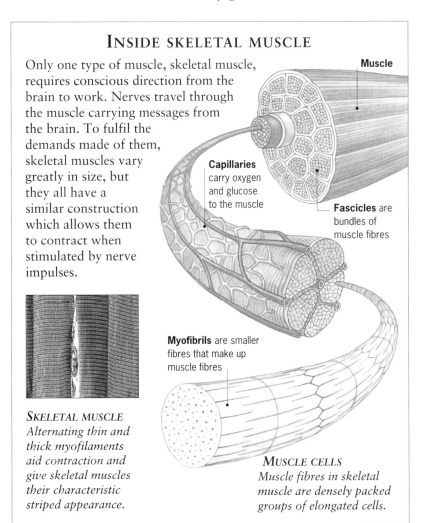

Muscle

Capillaries carry oxygen and glucose to the muscle

Fascicles are bundles of muscle fibres

Myofibrils are smaller fibres that make up muscle fibres

SKELETAL MUSCLE Alternating thin and thick myofilaments aid contraction and give skeletal muscles their characteristic striped appearance.

MUSCLE CELLS *Muscle fibres in skeletal muscle are densely packed groups of elongated cells.*

Pilates Instructor

Popular with dancers for more than 70 years, Pilates is now gaining in mainstream popularity as a form of exercise that improves overall body toning and posture as well as increasing flexibility without leaving you feeling exhausted.

A UNIVERSAL EXERCISE

Pilates first became popular with injured dancers who used the system to regain strength and flexibility. In fact, Pilates is beneficial for everyone regardless of age and physical strength.

▶ *Pregnant women can use Pilates throughout pregnancy and to help regain their shape after the birth.*

▶ *The system can be adapted to suit any age or condition.*

▶ *Pilates not only tones every muscle but can also aid weight loss. Half an hour of Pilates exercises burns 180–220 calories.*

Pilates (pronounced pih-lah-tees) is a system of exercise aimed at stretching, toning and balancing the whole body. Unlike weight training, the movements are fluid, rather than jerky, stretching muscles out to create sleekness rather than bulk. Instead of lifting weights or doing repetitions, the focus is on quality of specific movements and stretches. Pieces of equipment unique to the Pilates method are used to achieve this whole body toning.

What are the origins of Pilates?
In the early 1900s German-born Josef Pilates, an athlete who was also asthmatic, studied both Eastern and

THE PLIÉ MACHINE
Although it looks a bit like a medieval torture rack, the adjustable system of springs, straps and bars can stretch all the muscles of the body using the person's own body weight as resistance.

Western exercise systems to develop his own personal body-building programme. During the First World War, he worked as a nurse in England and experimented with attaching a system of springs to hospital beds to provide a way for patients to begin rehabilitation while still bedridden. This produced dramatic results and led him to go on to develop the Pilates system by inventing the plié machine (in America, where he first began teaching the system, it is known as the Universal Reformer). The method quickly became popular with professional dancers including famous names such as George Balanchine and Martha Graham.

What happens in a Pilates session?
Pilates training is usually done on a one-to-one basis, although some centres offer mat-work classes for advanced students. Before you begin, your instructor will probably analyse your postural needs looking at any areas of misalignment within the body. The session normally starts

with a warm-up, moving on to a series of floor exercises designed to strengthen the centre of the body (the muscles that circle the torso from the top of the hip bones to the base of the ribs). The floor work usually lasts around 30 minutes. After this, the session continues on the plié machine where every muscle of the legs can be worked, the back can be stretched and the arms built up. A beginner's programme would consist of a series of simple exercises lasting around 10 minutes (this can extend up to 45 minutes for the advanced). The upper body is then exercised with the use of free weights and equipment with names like 'the armchair' and 'the four-poster'. Individual postural requirements and physical needs are considered so that a tailormade session, unique to the Pilates method, can be followed.

How fit do I need to be?
The Pilates method lends itself to all levels of physical fitness and to all ages. As classes are choreographed for each individual, Pilates can provide a tough work-out for the fit and strong or a gentle stretching programme for less able individuals. Pilates is sometimes referred to as remedial gymnastics and physiotherapists and doctors frequently prescribe it. This is because Pilates can work around injured areas giving the surrounding areas a thorough work-out. It can also be used as a method of rehabilitation increasing strength and flexibility once an injury has healed.

How quickly will I see results?
You will 'feel' different after just one session – lighter, more balanced and taller. Many people report feeling energised, which sets the method apart from some work-outs which leave you feeling exhausted. For the best results, as with any exercise, regular continued practice is necessary. As it is an exercise which you can do at any age, if it suits you, there's no need to stop, at any point. Many

professional dancers and, in recent years, even rugby players, have extended their careers by using the method.

What training do Pilates practitioners have?
There are several Pilates Associations in the UK where qualified practitioners are certified. They will already have trained in another field such as dance, gymnastics, sport, physiotherapy or medicine before learning Pilates. Pilates training combines background knowledge of physiology and anatomy with several years' practical training in the Pilates method.

Can Pilates help particular health problems?
The Pilates method can help the nervous system, easing migraine, tension headache, depression, seasonal affective disorder, and the metabolism. Pilates promotes healthy cardiovascular, respiratory and digestive systems, and can relieve complaints of the musculoskeletal system, such as lumbar/sacral disc problems, knee pain, and pressure on cartilage or joints. Regular controlled exercise can help to lower high blood pressure and problems with the urogenital system such as stress incontinence which can be relieved.

WHAT YOU CAN DO AT HOME

Once you are familiar with the Pilates way of moving and your body has improved in flexibility, there will be a number of exercises you can practise at home in between Pilates sessions. These exercises usually concentrate on building strength in the abdominal region.

The exercise shown here is called 'the rolling ball' and is intended to

be performed in one slow and controlled continuous movement. If your abdominals aren't strong enough to take you from the end of step 2 back to the starting position, it may help to build some momentum by gently rocking back and forth. If you feel happy with the exercise perform it for 5–10 repetitions three times a week.

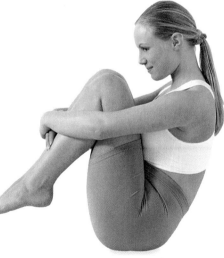

1 *Sit up with your knees bent and pulled tight into your chest. Wrap your arms around your legs with your hands on your shins. Bring your nose towards your knees, rounding your spine slightly into a C-shape as you lift your toes off the mat, balancing on your buttocks.*

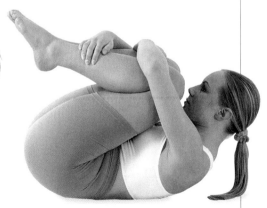

2 *Using your abdominal muscles, slowly roll backwards to balance on your middle back and shoulder blades, without altering the position of your arms and legs. In a continuous movement, roll forwards to the start position. Keep your heels close to your buttocks.*

called myofibrils. These house even smaller filaments, actin and myosin, which are responsible for muscular contraction (see page 80). The actin and myosin filaments are divided up along the length of the muscle filament into sections called sarcomeres. Under a microscope, actin is seen as a thin line while myosin is thicker and darker. The alternation of these two filaments gives skeletal muscle a distinctive striated – or striped – appearance.

When the muscle is stimulated to contract by a signal from the nervous system, the actin and myosin filaments draw towards each other like fingers being interlaced. This results in the shortening of the myofibrils, muscle fibres, and, consequently, the overall muscle length.

Connective tissue

Throughout the body there are various types of fibrous connective tissue, or fascia. In particular, fascia is found extensively within the muscles where it reduces friction between their various components as well as carrying nerves, blood and lymphatic

vessels. Each muscle has three separate layers of fascia. These layers extend from the ends of the muscles to form dense lengths of connective tissue called tendons, which mainly attach muscles to bones. In some places the muscles are attached to other muscles via a broad flat tendon known as an aponeurosis.

A characteristic that is common to all tendons is their relative lack of elasticity. They have far less potential to stretch than muscles and so are vulnerable to injury, especially when cold.

Ligaments, like tendons, are also made of dense connective tissue and are designed to give extra support to the joints. Ligaments also have a limited degree of pliability in order to allow the joint to move, but they are positioned so as to prevent the joint from moving outside its intended range. If the ligaments were too elastic, the joints would be too unstable to allow normal controlled movement. Overstretching the ligaments is a common cause of weak joints, especially the ankles.

Connective tissue is greatly affected by temperature, becoming much more pliable when warm. A controlled programme of gentle exercises and stretches that warm up the muscles and joints prior to vigorous exercise will reduce the likelihood of injury and enhance flexibility.

BUILDING MUSCLE

When muscles are regularly called on to cope with a heavier load than they had previously been used to, they respond to the extra demand by increasing the number of

TENDONS AND LIGAMENTS OF THE HAND

Both ligaments and tendons are made up of dense fibres of connective tissue called collagen – a tough, flexible protein. The ligaments support bones, mainly in and around joints, to allow controlled movements and prevent the joint from overextending. Tendons provide a strong link between skeletal muscle and bone. Those in the hand extend up the arm to their controlling muscles situated near the elbow.

The retinaculum is a thick band of ligament tissue positioned to give the wrist stability and prevent it from moving beyond its range

Tendons react to the contraction of muscle by moving a bone at a joint

Subcutaneous fat

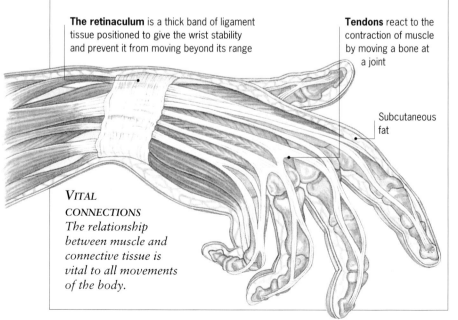

VITAL CONNECTIONS
The relationship between muscle and connective tissue is vital to all movements of the body.

HOW MUSCLES GUARD AGAINST DAMAGE

The brain sends commands to the muscles via the motor nerves of the central nervous system. The initial effects of resistance training mainly occur within these nerve pathways as the body learns to stimulate

muscle fibres in the correct sequence to accomplish the movement. Muscles guard against damage by automatically reducing their work output or stopping in the face of fatigue. This is called the principle of inhibition.

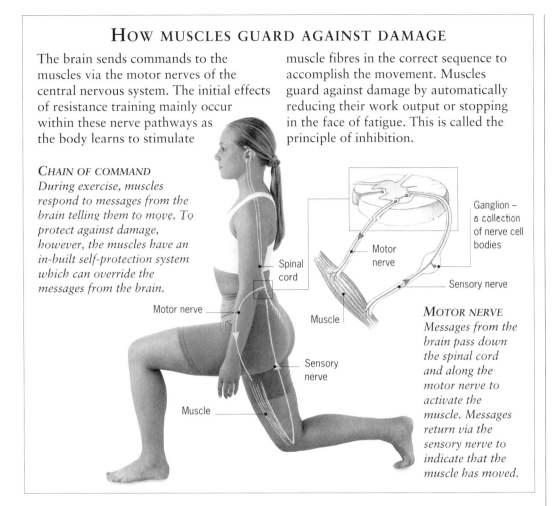

CHAIN OF COMMAND
During exercise, muscles respond to messages from the brain telling them to move. To protect against damage, however, the muscles have an in-built self-protection system which can override the messages from the brain.

Ganglion – a collection of nerve cell bodies

Motor nerve

Spinal cord

Sensory nerve

Muscle

Motor nerve

Sensory nerve

Muscle

MOTOR NERVE
Messages from the brain pass down the spinal cord and along the motor nerve to activate the muscle. Messages return via the sensory nerve to indicate that the muscle has moved.

myofilaments inside the muscle cells. This causes an increase in the tone and size of the muscle, known as hypertrophy, and so strengthens the muscles.

The way that muscles respond to different forms of exercise is determined by the different types of fibre. Muscles contain three types of fibre: slow-twitch, fast-twitch and intermediate-twitch fibres. Slow-twitch fibres are thin fibres with a plentiful supply of capillary blood vessels. They also contain a large store of myoglobin, which increases their oxygen supply, and numerous mitochondria (see page 59), structures where aerobic energy production occurs. Their primary source of fuel is fat which, with their rich oxygen supply, gives them a high endurance level. This means they can carry out low-intensity tasks for long periods of time, providing oxygen can be supplied to meet their needs. However, their narrow size limits their power and intensity.

Fast-twitch fibres are double the width of slow-twitch fibres. They have large reserves of glycogen but are poorly supplied with

blood capillaries and mitochondria, so are powered by anaerobic energy systems. Because of their large size they can contract in a sudden, powerful way to overcome high resistance, requiring no oxygen to do so. But they lack endurance and tire quickly.

Intermediate-twitch fibres are between the other two types in size, so are more powerful than slow-twitch fibres. They are well supplied with capillaries and mitochondria and so are powered by the aerobic system, giving them a degree of endurance, but not as much as slow-twitch fibres.

All muscles contain a mixture of these fibres, but in varying proportions, depending on the muscle's function. Partly for genetic reasons, but also in response to training, some people have more of some types of fibres than others. The leg muscles of marathon runners have 80 per cent slow and intermediate-twitch fibres, whereas sprinters' leg muscles have 60 per cent fast-twitch fibres. Weightlifters' legs have an equal mixture of fast and slow/intermediate-twitch fibres.

MUSCLE INTELLIGENCE
In training, a long-distance runner focuses on muscular endurance and long-term energy release from the muscles. The muscles respond to regular training by increasing in slow-twitch fibres which have a high endurance level. If the person were to give up long-distance running and take up sprinting instead, the muscles would respond by increasing in fast-twitch fibres which are more powerful for high-intensity work.

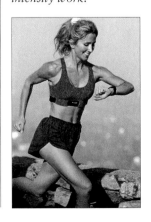

An exercise overview
The American College of Sports Medicine recommends that for health benefits people should do resistance training twice a week. They suggest that each session should take a whole body approach including 8 to 12 exercises for the various major muscle groups. It is not only muscles that become stronger with strength training but also tendons, ligaments and bones.

Slow-twitch and intermediate-twitch fibres respond to training by improving their ability to utilise oxygen. Regular endurance training increases the number of capillaries, which enhances their ability to transport carbon dioxide and oxygen. The mitochondria also increase in number and size. The overall effect is enhanced muscle tone. Fast-twitch fibres have the potential to bulk up with high-intensity resistance training.

Whether an exercise programme achieves increases in muscle size or simply enhances muscle tone depends on whether training focuses on resistance work or endurance.

Regular exercise makes the muscle fibres more efficient, so fewer muscle fibres are needed for any given strength exercise. This leaves others free to take over when they become exhausted. Such economy of effort means that work can be continued for longer, producing endurance benefits.

Building and toning

The term muscle building suggests the development of greater muscle mass, and it is possible to design a training programme that will result in larger muscles. But it is also possible to become stronger, and to improve endurance, without substantially increasing the size of muscle.

Many women avoid strength training because they worry about developing a masculine-looking body. But unless a woman is born with an above average number of fast-twitch fibres and abnormal levels of the male hormone testosterone, which aids muscle building, and then trains diligently at high intensities, she is unlikely to produce abnormal muscle bulk.

As the body responds in very specific ways, according to how it is challenged, a programme of resistance training can be designed to achieve either muscular bulk or simply a heightened state of tone.

To bring about improvements in muscle strength or endurance, muscles must be regularly challenged to work at a level just beyond their present capabilities. This is known as applying overload. To increase strength the muscle must overcome progressively greater resistance, whereas to improve endurance it is the duration of the exercise that is gradually extended. The ways that muscles adapt in response to overload are called the training effects.

Improving muscle tone without increasing bulk

To improve muscle tone, without significantly increasing muscle bulk, exercises need to focus on challenging the slow-twitch fibres. This is done by working with levels of resistance that are moderate enough to allow many repetitions.

Because of the low endurance capabilities of fast-twitch fibres, strength work involves a few repetitions repeated several times in groups, or sets, with rest or recovery periods between each set.

In comparison, endurance training focuses on the slow and intermediate fibres and so uses lower levels of resistance. It involves fewer sets, but a higher number of consecutive repetitions thereby challenging the stamina of the muscles. When designing your own programme, in order to improve your shape remember the benefits of strength work as well as endurance training.

EVERYDAY MUSCLE USAGE

Many of our muscles get used at some point during the day, just some of which are listed here. Due to increasingly sedentary lives, however, many muscles are underworked. When we then perform out-of-the-ordinary tasks, such as mowing the lawn or decorating, underworked muscles can become quickly fatigued.

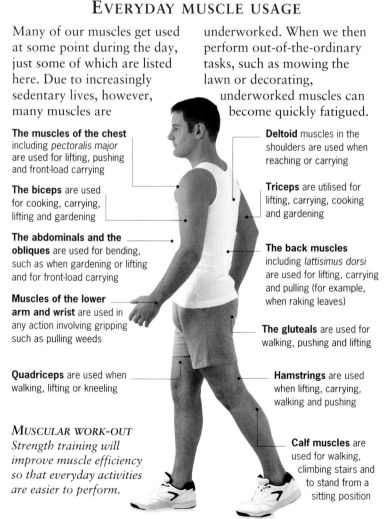

The muscles of the chest including *pectoralis major* are used for lifting, pushing and front-load carrying

The biceps are used for cooking, carrying, lifting and gardening

The abdominals and the obliques are used for bending, such as when gardening or lifting and for front-load carrying

Muscles of the lower arm and wrist are used in any action involving gripping such as pulling weeds

Quadriceps are used when walking, lifting or kneeling

Deltoid muscles in the shoulders are used when reaching or carrying

Triceps are utilised for lifting, carrying, cooking and gardening

The back muscles including *lattisimus dorsi* are used for lifting, carrying and pulling (for example, when raking leaves)

The gluteals are used for walking, pushing and lifting

Hamstrings are used when lifting, carrying, walking and pushing

Calf muscles are used for walking, climbing stairs and to stand from a sitting position

MUSCULAR WORK-OUT
Strength training will improve muscle efficiency so that everyday activities are easier to perform.

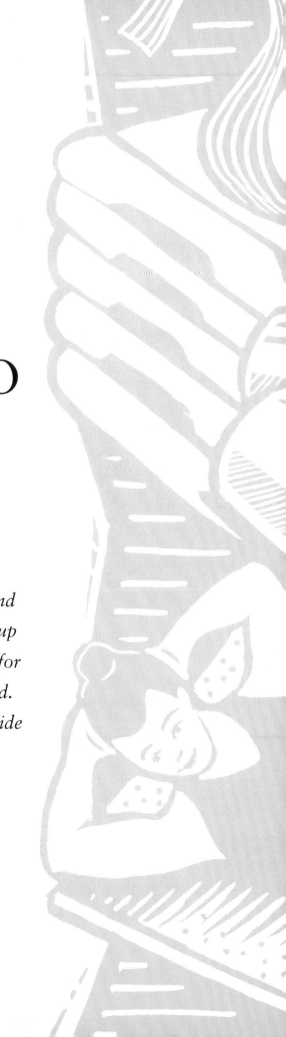

CHAPTER 5

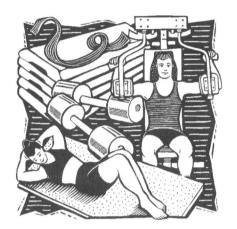

EXERCISES TO SHAPE UP YOUR BODY

This chapter provides step-by-step photographs and instructions for exercises to strengthen and shape up your whole body. Each exercise is safe to perform for most people, from beginners to the more advanced. Tables at the beginning of the chapter provide a guide to the number of times each exercise should be performed according to your level of fitness.

BEGINNING TO EXERCISE

Embarking on an exercise programme need not be daunting. Over the following pages you will find a comprehensive package of exercises designed to develop strength, tone and flexibility.

If you play a sport, or just want to gain an all-round improvement in your strength and shape, this chapter will show you how the different muscle groups in your body work, and the best way to tone and strengthen them. If you wish to improve a particular part of your body, either because it has been weakened through injury or suffered from lack of use, or you want to strengthen yourself in order to perform a particular task or play a sport better, this chapter will show you exercises to help you to achieve your goal.

HOW TO USE THIS CHAPTER

The exercises which appear on the following pages have been organised according to the different muscle groups of the body, beginning with the head and neck. Most of the exercises can easily be performed at home with no special equipment. However, some useful exercises using machines found in gyms have also been included.

To shape up your whole body, work through the chapter, performing each set of exercises methodically. The exercises are designed for both men and women to perform. Although people often want different results from an exercise programme – men often want to look and feel stronger, whereas women usually want to become firmer and slimmer – the means of achieving these goals are much the same. The charts on pages 96 and 97 provide a general guide to the number of times you should perform each exercise depending on your level of fitness; however, remember it's important to establish your basic level of fitness before starting any kind of exercise programme.

Before beginning any of the exercises shown, make sure that you warm up thoroughly. This is of particular importance if you are stretching your muscles or using weights. If you do not warm up first you could tear a muscle or cause another type of painful and debilitating injury. Walk or jog on the spot for at least five minutes to get your body moving. While you are walking, swing your arms and loosen your joints. Begin your warm-up slowly, gradually increasing the level of exertion as you continue, and this will help you to avoid much of the stiffness many people experience the day after taking some exercise.

Each section of the chapter begins with an illustration of the main muscles in the section of the body being addressed and a description of some common shape problems. Basic stretches are shown before the

RESISTANCE EQUIPMENT

Although you can perform most exercises effectively without any special equipment, in some instances – and particularly if you are at the intermediate or advanced level – dumbbells, wrist and ankle weights and an elastic band may be very helpful. Wrist and ankle weights can be worn while performing more active forms of exercise to provide a greater challenge, while elastic bands and dumbbells will help you to develop greater strength and tone during controlled exercise. All these items can be bought at sports stores, or you can use them free of charge at the gym.

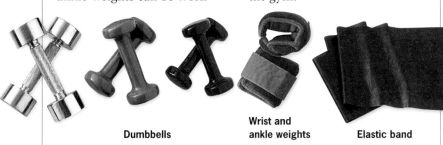

Dumbbells

Wrist and ankle weights

Elastic band

exercises. It is important to perform these first in order to allow your muscles to get used to the movement before you begin toning in earnest. It is also important to cool down after exercising, especially if you have pushed yourself hard. Relax by doing some gentle stretches then treat yourself to a soothing aromatherapy bath.

Each muscle in the body works as part of a pair (see page 80). This is why it is important to complete the whole of an exercise to ensure that each partner within the pair is strengthened equally. If one muscle becomes strong through a great deal of use, its com-

panion muscle could become weaker, bunched up and ultimately cause posture problems and pain. You should also try to ensure that your body is strengthened equally. If you have one area that is weak, others may compensate for it and you could find yourself in pain.

Finally, if you suffer from any medical condition, such as heart disease, diabetes or you are pregnant, make sure you consult your doctor before you begin exercising. There may be exercises that you should avoid, or exercises that could be particularly beneficial to your health.

THE MAIN MUSCLES OF THE BODY

There are over 600 muscles in the human body, each one working as part of a pair to allow the body sufficient strength and flexibility to carry out everyday activities. Skeletal muscles are attached to bones and cross joints, providing them with the force to move. Muscles are layered in the body, and often overlap each other. Those that are just below the skin are known as superficial muscles, and beneath them are the deep muscles. With proper use of the body, all the muscles are used. The larger muscles and the ones most commonly targeted by exercise programmes are shown here.

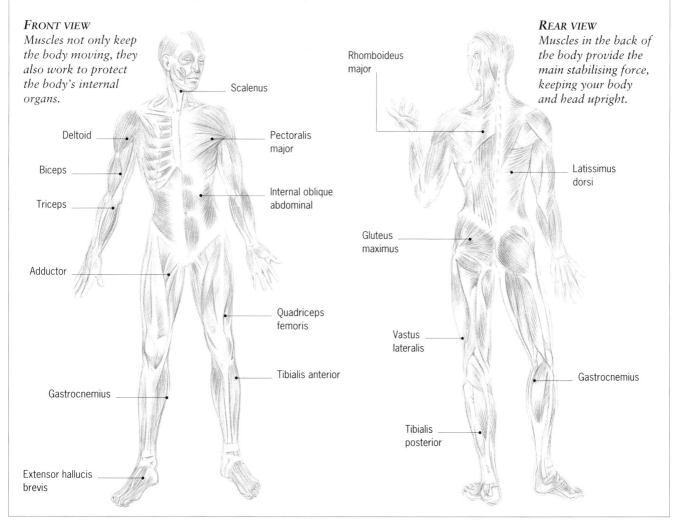

FRONT VIEW
Muscles not only keep the body moving, they also work to protect the body's internal organs.

Scalenus
Deltoid
Biceps
Triceps
Pectoralis major
Internal oblique abdominal
Adductor
Quadriceps femoris
Tibialis anterior
Gastrocnemius
Extensor hallucis brevis

REAR VIEW
Muscles in the back of the body provide the main stabilising force, keeping your body and head upright.

Rhomboideus major
Latissimus dorsi
Gluteus maximus
Vastus lateralis
Gastrocnemius
Tibialis posterior

A General Exercise Programme

One of the most important aspects of beginning an exercise programme is establishing clear and realistic short and long-term goals in order to maintain motivation and help you to measure improvements. The four programmes below provide a general guide for building strength, tone and mobility for every level of fitness over a 12-week period.

In order to choose the correct exercise programme for you, take your resting pulse rate (see page 86) which gives a general idea of your basic level of fitness. Each programme is designed to work all the main muscle groups. Follow each exercise in the order shown in the chart. 'Reps' refers to the number of times to perform the movement while the set is the total number of repetitions. Allow a 30-second rest between each set. Follow the programme at least twice a week, and include a warm-up and stretches before and after exercising.

BEGINNER'S PROGRAMME

		WEEKS 1-4			WEEKS 5-8			WEEKS 9-12		
BODY PART	EXERCISE	SETS	REPS	WEIGHT	SETS	REPS	WEIGHT	SETS	REPS	WEIGHT
Chest	Press-up easy	1	10-20	-	2	10-20	-	3	10-20	-
Back	Seated row with band	1	10-20	-	2	10-20	-	3	10-20	-
	Superman	1	10-20	-	2	10-20	-	3	10-20	-
Shoulders	Dumbbell lateral raise	1	10-20	-	2	10-20	-	3	10-20	-
Legs	Squat	1	10-20	-	2	10-20	-	3	10-20	-
	Inner thigh	1	10-20	-	2	10-20	-	3	10-20	-
	Outer thigh	1	10-20	-	2	10-20	-	3	10-20	-
Abdominals	Basic crunch	1	10-20	-	2	10-20	-	3	10-20	-
	Oblique curl	1	10-20	-	2	10-20	-	3	10-20	-

INTERMEDIATE PROGRAMME

		WEEKS 1-4			WEEKS 5-8			WEEKS 9-12		
BODY PART	EXERCISE	SETS	REPS	WEIGHT	SETS	REPS	WEIGHT	SETS	REPS	WEIGHT
Chest	Press-up easy	2	10-20	-	3	10-20	-	3	10-20	-
	Flat bench or incline flyes	1	10-20	-	2	10-20	-	3	10-20	-
Back	Seated row with band	2	10-20	-	3	10-20	-	3	10-20	-
	Superman	2	10-20	-	2	10-20	-	3	10-20	-
	Reverse flyes	1	10-20	-	2	10-20	-	3	10-20	-
Shoulders and	Dumbbell lateral raise	2	10-20	-	3	10-20	-	3	10-20	-
arms	Triceps dip easy	1	10-20	-	2	10-20	-	3	10-20	-
	Concentration curls	1	10-20	-	2	10-20	-	3	10-20	-
Legs	Squat	3	10-20	-	3	10-20	-	3	10-20	-
	Inner thigh	2	10-20	-	3	10-20	-	3	10-20	-
	Outer thigh	2	10-20	-	3	10-20	-	3	10-20	-
	Glute lift	1	10-20	-	2	10-20	-	3	10-20	-
Abdominals	Basic crunch	3	10-20	-	3	10-20	-	3	10-20	-
	Pelvic flattening	3	10-20	-	3	10-20	-	3	10-20	-
	Alternating leg kicks	1	10-20	-	2	10-20	-	3	10-20	-
	Oblique curl	1	10-20	-	2	10-20	-	3	10-20	-

ADVANCED PROGRAMME

BODY PART	EXERCISE	WEEKS 1 -4			WEEKS 5 -8			WEEKS 9 -12		
		SETS	REPS	WEIGHT	SETS	REPS	WEIGHT	SETS	REPS	WEIGHT
Chest	Press-up easy/advanced	3	10-20	-	3	10-20	-	3	10-20	-
	Flat bench or incline flyes	2	10-20	-	3	10-20	-	3	10-20	-
	Flat dumbbell press	1	10-20	-	2	10-20	-	3	10-20	-
Back	Seated row with band	3	10-20	-	3	10-20	-	3	10-20	-
	Superman	3	10-20	-	3	10-20	-	3	10-20	-
	Reverse flyes	2	10-20	-	3	10-20	-	3	10-20	-
	Single arm row	1	10-20	-	2	10-20	-	3	10-20	-
Shoulders and arms	Dumbbell shoulder press	1	10-20	-	2	10-20	-	3	10-20	-
	Dumbbell lateral raise	2	10-20	-	3	10-20	-	3	10-20	-
	Triceps dip easy/advanced	3	10-20	-	3	10-20	-	3	10-20	-
	Concentration curls	3	10-20	-	3	10-20	-	3	10-20	-
Legs	Squat	2	10-20	-	3	10-20	-	3	10-20	-
	Lunge – single leg	1	10-20	-	2	10-20	-	3	10-20	-
	Inner thigh	3	10-20	-	3	10-20	-	3	10-20	-
	Outer thigh	3	10-20	-	3	10-20	-	3	10-20	-
	Glute lift	3	10-20	-	3	10-20	-	3	10-20	-
Abdominals	Basic crunch/advanced	2	10-20	-	3	10-20	-	3	10-20	-
	Pelvic flattening	3	10-20	-	3	10-20	-	3	10-20	-
	Alternating leg kicks	3	10-20	-	3	10-20	-	3	10-20	-
	Oblique curl/advanced	2	10-20	-	2	10-20	-	3	10-20	-

GENERAL MOBILITY PROGRAMME

Many people neglect their general flexibility when developing an exercise programme, but good flexibility is vital for overall mobility and ease of movement. As you age, or if your occupation is primarily sedentary, you may find your muscles weaken and shorten. This can lead to stiffness and aches and pains that can seriously limit your general level of activity and ability. Performing the programme below regularly should help you to maintain good strength and flexibility. Remember, if you suffer from arthritis or any other serious joint or bone disorder, you must discuss your exercise plans with your doctor first.

BODY PART	EXERCISE	WEEKS 1 -4			WEEKS 5 -8			WEEKS 9 -12		
		SETS	REPS	WEIGHT	SETS	REPS	WEIGHT	SETS	REPS	WEIGHT
Neck	Head rotation	1	10	-	2	10	-	3	10	-
	Deep neck flexor	1	10-20	-	2	10-20	-	3	10-20	-
	Upper trapezius stretch	-	1			2		-	3	-
	Scalene stretch	-	1			2		-	3	-
Hands	Wrist mobility exercise	1	10-20	-	2	10-20	-	3	10-20	-
	Wrist strengthening – ball	1	10-20	-	2	10-20	-	3	10-20	-
	Wrist extensor stretch	-	1		-	2		-	3	-
	Wrist flexor stretch	-	1		-	2		-	3	-
Feet	Arch exercise	1	10-20	-	2	10-20	-	3	10-20	-
	Foot dorsi flexion	1	10-20	-	2	10-20	-	3	10-20	-
	Toe extensor stretch	-	1		-	2		-	3	

Head and Neck

The muscles of the head and neck are often neglected in exercise programmes. Regularly exercising and stretching these muscles can help to avoid muscular pain, fatigue and headaches and reduce the risk of developing arthritis.

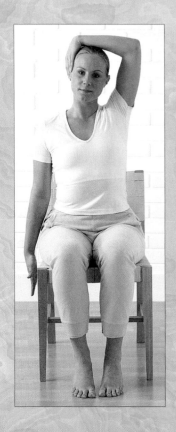

COMPLEMENTARY NECK EXERCISE

▶ Yoga is an excellent form of exercise for the neck muscles. Many yoga postures require extensive stretching and muscle strength.

▶ Because water supports the weight of the head, swimming and aqua-aerobics provide a safe environment in which to extend the neck muscles through a wide range of movement.

The numerous muscles of the face usually get enough exercise from the range of normal facial expressions to maintain adequate tone. There is an important group of muscles that move the head and cervical spine, however, that do require regular toning exercise.

The sternocleidomastoids (SCM) are two prominent and powerful muscles at the front and sides of the neck. They are attached to the top of the breastbone and the collarbone and are connected to the skull, just below the ear. Their main actions are to pull the head to the side (lateral flexion) and rotate the head in the opposite direction. Both SCMs work together to lift the head from a prone position and to help to lift the chest during heavy exertion. In adults the head weighs about 5 kg (11 lbs), so the SCMs need to be fairly strong.

The SCM muscle can be felt easily: place your left index finger on the end of your left collarbone (which is in the hollow of the throat). Now turn your head slowly to your right and you will feel the SCM push against your finger as it contracts.

The scalenes are joined to the front of the neck (cervical) vertebra and attached to the first rib. These muscles can bend the neck forwards (flexion), and to the side (lateral flexion) and rotate the head to the opposite side. The scalenes also aid respiration during heavy exertion by lifting the first rib, allowing more space for the lungs to expand.

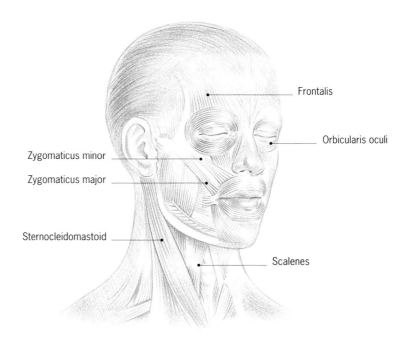

Frontalis

Orbicularis oculi

Zygomaticus minor

Zygomaticus major

Sternocleidomastoid

Scalenes

Exercises to target the neck

Performing stretching exercises to increase flexibility and strength in the neck and facial muscles can make a difference to the rest of your work-out. Many people's upper bodies are very stiff and tense, causing headaches and excessive tiredness at the end of the day. Increasing the suppleness of your neck muscles can greatly improve your energy levels.

NECK STRETCHES

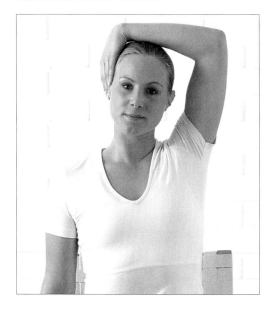

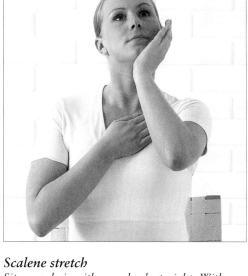

Don't allow your lower back to overarch. This places stress on the vertebrae of the lower back and may cause pain.

Don't let your head fall backwards. This places stress on the vertebrae at the back of the neck.

Upper trapezius stretch
Sit on a chair with your back upright and shoulders level. Ease your left hand towards the floor with fingers pointing down. Rest your right hand over the left ear and ease your head slightly to the right until a mild stretch is felt. Hold for 10–30 seconds, breathing evenly. Slowly release. and repeat on the other side.

Scalene stretch
Sit on a chair with your back straight. With your right hand, support your chin in a slightly upright position. Rest your left hand on your sternum. Rotate your head slightly to the left. Look up and depress the sternum with your left hand so a mild stretch is felt. Hold for 10–30 seconds. Release and repeat on the other side.

Head rotation
This exercise stretches the SCM and scalenes. Sit in a chair with your back upright. Slowly turn your head to one side, stopping as soon as you feel a mild stretch. Hold for 10 seconds, return to start position and stretch the other side. Repeat 5–10 times.

Deep neck extensors
Ensure you are sitting in a low-backed rigid chair before starting this exercise.

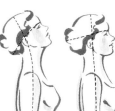 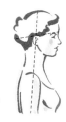 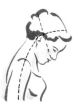 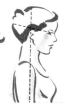 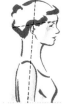

1. Begin by tilting your head back slightly

2. Draw your chin forwards and level your head

3. Keeping your head level, return to upright

4. Tilt your chin towards your chest

5. Ease your head backwards, keeping chin down

6. Finish by slowly raising your chin and head back to upright

The Chest

Your chest shape can be determined by many factors: your body type, diet, the amount and type of exercise you perform and your posture are all critical. There is much you can do to improve your chest shape with specific strengthening exercises.

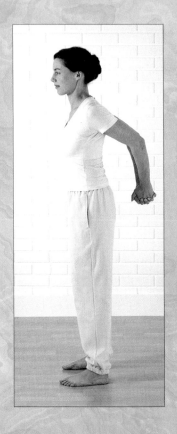

The chest muscles can be a source of shape problems for both men and women. Typically, men may be concerned about weak chest muscles, or a 'sunken' appearance, while many women worry about their breast shape. However, strong chest muscles are important for everyone: we all need to maintain a certain amount of strength for everyday lifting and carrying, and good chest function may also improve posture, relieve aches and pains, and in turn improve the efficiency of the lungs.

The anatomy of the chest

The large pectoral muscle (pectoralis major) is the biggest and most powerful muscle of the chest. This triangular muscle is joined to the upper torso in two places: a small portion is connected to the collarbone (clavicle), while the largest part is linked to the breast bone (sternum). All the fibres of the muscle converge into a flat tendon that is attached to the upper arm bone (humerus). In women, a large portion of the

COMPLEMENTARY CHEST EXERCISE

▶ Swimming, especially breaststroke, the crawl and butterfly promote strong pectorals.

▶ The reaching shots in racquet sports require and enhance strong pectorals.

▶ Posture can make a huge difference to your chest shape. The Alexander technique can help you improve rounded shoulders or a weak back.

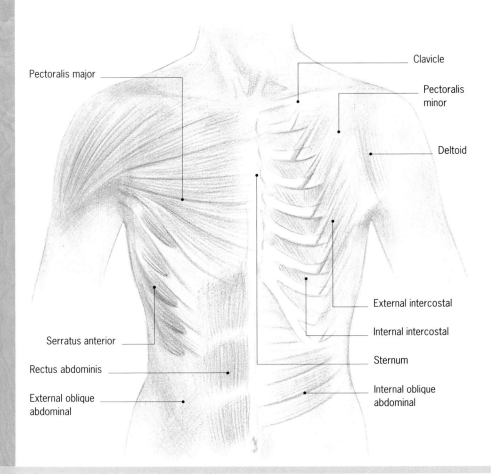

Pectoralis major

Clavicle

Pectoralis minor

Deltoid

External intercostal

Internal intercostal

Serratus anterior

Rectus abdominis

Sternum

External oblique abdominal

Internal oblique abdominal

breast overlies this muscle. The main action of the pectoralis major is to draw the arm across the front of the body, a movement known as adduction. The whole of the muscle can be made to contract by placing the hands together in front of the body and pressing them together. The pectoralis major is in two main parts that often work independently and so are sometimes referred to as the 'upper' and 'lower' pectoral muscles. During heavy exertion, the whole muscle may also be used to aid breathing.

Another muscle, the anterior deltoid, works with the pectoralis major in many movements. Its principal role is to lift the arm forwards from the side of the body, an action called flexion.

Underneath the pectoral muscle is a smaller triangular muscle called the pectoralis minor. This is linked to the third, fourth and fifth ribs and the shoulder blade. It moves the shoulder blade forwards and down, and also acts as a stabiliser.

Chest problems

Like any other muscle, the chest muscles will weaken with lack of use: for men this can lead to sagging pectorals. Specific strength exercises will tone the pectorals and over time restore their firmness, but it is important to look at diet issues in conjunction with exercise. Cutting back on high-fat foods will also do much to improve shape.

Breast problems

The breasts lie over the muscles of the chest and are mainly composed of fat; therefore exercises aimed at changing breast size may have limited success. When a women has large breasts and excess body fat, a programme designed to reduce overall body fat levels will often lead to a reduction in breast size too. All women, however, benefit from exercises to tone the pectoral muscles underlying the breasts.

SHAPE CHALLENGE
Sagging breasts

With age many women experience the problem of a loss of breast firmness. This can be particularly noticeable after beginning breastfeeding. Unfortunately, because of the anatomy of the breast, this can be a difficult problem to overcome. The firmness of the breasts is dependent on the suspensory ligaments (see page 71). These ligaments are non-elastic, and once stretched by, for example, significant weight gain, cannot be restored to their original size. However, exercise and diet can do much to improve your breast shape and strengthen the chest muscle below the breast.

CASE HISTORY

Suzy is a 37-year-old woman with a 12-month-old son, Paul. Since weaning Paul six months ago she has been keen to restore her breasts to their former shape, but has had little success. She has begun attending weekly aerobics classes, and has tried to cut back on high-fat foods. However, although she has lost some weight generally, she is still unhappy with her breast size and shape.

Suzy's regime

▶ *Suzy needs to perform exercises particularly targeted towards the chest muscles. By toning the pectorals supporting the breasts she should gain a fuller breast shape. Exercises that are particularly suitable are the pec dec, incline chest press and flyes.*

▶ *To maintain Suzy's general level of fitness but better target her chest muscles, she should take up a sport such as tennis or swimming.*

SHAPE CHALLENGE
A sunken chest

Some men develop a flat-chested or 'sunken' physique in which the abdomen protrudes farther than the chest. This is usually due to lack of tone in the pectoral muscles. The appearance is worsened when there is excess body fat around the abdominal area. Young men should remember that they will continue to develop physically until the age of about 25, so an 18-year-old's expectations of a well-developed chest may be unrealistic. With some attention to exercise and diet, however, major improvements in shape and strength can be achieved relatively easily.

CASE HISTORY

Tony is a 20-year-old student unhappy with his lack of chest development. He eats plenty of food but hardly ever seems to put on weight in the right areas, and is finding his abdomen is better defined than his chest. Tony thinks he gets plenty of exercise as he is a keen footballer, playing for his college. He is aware he possibly drinks too much, but thinks he should be 'burning off' most of his calories.

Tony's regime

▶ *Tony would benefit from some specific chest strengthening exercises. Because he is young and fit he should be able to perform 20 press-ups three times a week. Purchasing some dumbbells could also help him to reach his shape goals faster.*

▶ *Tony's diet could be improved by cutting back on high-fat food. This would prevent him storing excess fat around his stomach.*

Exercises to target the chest

Tight, restricted chest muscles can contribute to a round-shouldered posture so it is important that the pectoral muscles are stretched regularly. Because the pectoralis major runs in three different directions, a number of different stretches and exercises should be performed to strengthen the muscle as a whole. Many of these exercises also work other muscles in the upper body such as the deltoid at the shoulder joint.

CHEST AND SHOULDER STRETCHES

Stand tall with feet hip-width apart. Lock your fingers together behind your back, contract the abdominals and soften the knees. To perform the stretch, gently ease the elbows up and away from the body until you can feel the stretch across the chest and shoulders. Try not to lean forwards. Hold for 20–30 seconds, breathing easily.

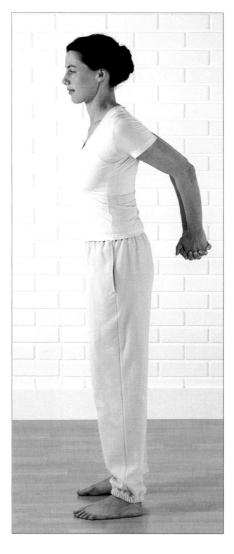

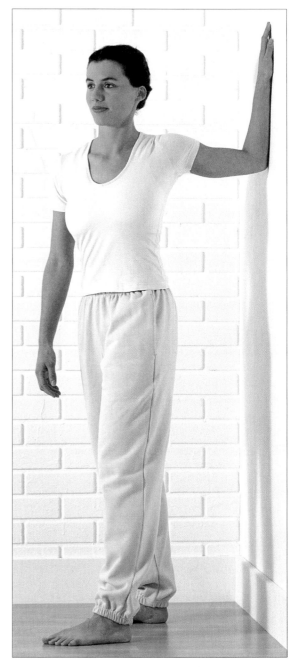

Deep stretch ▶
Place the palm of your hand flat against a wall with the arm at right angles to your body. Rotate your body away from the arm until a stretch is felt in the chest and front of the shoulder. Hold for 20–30 seconds, breathing easily. Change arms.

PRESS-UPS: *Works pectorals, front deltoids, triceps*

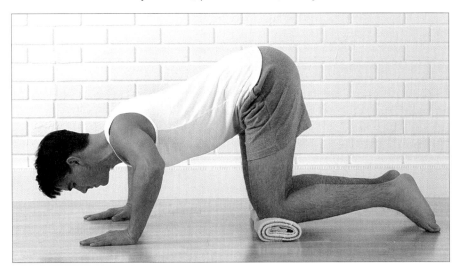

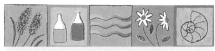

ALMOND OIL

One of the most important of the natural moisturisers is almond oil. It is extracted from the oil-enriched kernels of sweet, ripe almonds. You can add it to moisturisers or use it as a massage oil.

To make a gentle exfoliator for the tender skin of the breasts mix 25 g (1 oz) of ground oatmeal with the same amount of finely ground almonds and add 15 ml (1 tbsp) of almond oil. Massage gently into the breasts and then rinse thoroughly.

Beginner's easy press-up
Start on your hands and knees. If necessary, rest your knees on a mat for comfort. Your hands should be positioned facing forwards, under your shoulders.

Keep your abdominals contracted. Bend your elbows and lower your chest to the floor slowly, inhaling on the way down. Press up to start position, exhaling. Timing: 4 seconds down, 4 seconds up.

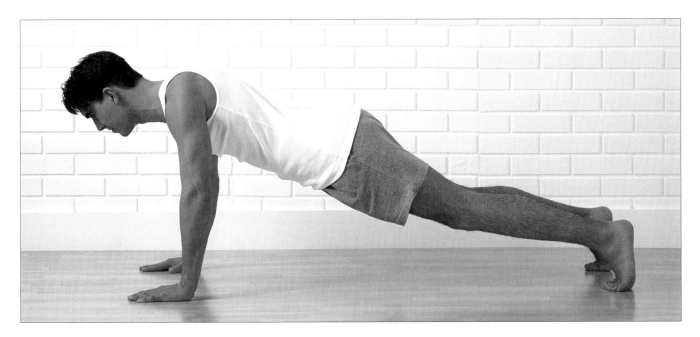

Advanced press-up
To increase the intensity of the beginner's press-up, come up from your knees onto your toes, distributing your weight over your hands and feet. Place your feet a little wider apart to help with your balance if required. With abdominals contracted, bend your elbows out 90° and lower your chest towards the floor, inhaling. Press back up to the starting position, exhaling.

Don't let your abdominals sag, as this places stress on the vertebrae of the lower back and can lead to injury. Keep your back straight at all times.

Don't lift your head up too high. This places strain on the neck and can also result in injury.

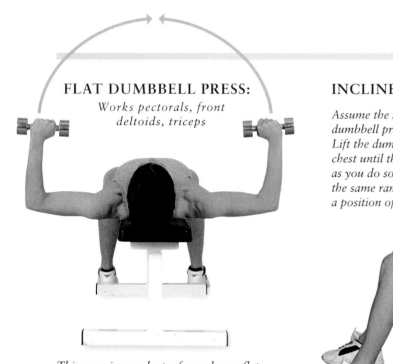

FLAT DUMBBELL PRESS:

Works pectorals, front deltoids, triceps

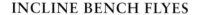

This exercise can be performed on a flat or inclined bench. Inclining the bench will make the exercise slightly easier. Keep the abdominals contracted and lower your back flat onto a bench or step. Assume the starting position as shown above with arms bent at 90° to your body. Lift the dumbbells in an arc above your chest until they almost touch. Return to the start position.

INCLINE DUMBBELL PRESS

Assume the start position as for the flat dumbbell press but on an incline bench. Lift the dumbbells in an arc above your chest until they almost touch, exhaling as you do so. Lower the weights through the same range, inhaling. Only lower to a position of mild stretch.

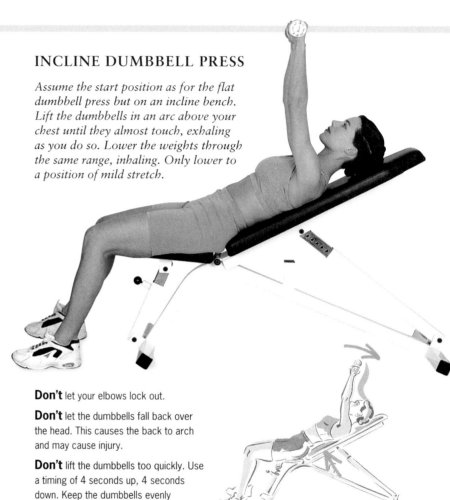

Don't let your elbows lock out.

Don't let the dumbbells fall back over the head. This causes the back to arch and may cause injury.

Don't lift the dumbbells too quickly. Use a timing of 4 seconds up, 4 seconds down. Keep the dumbbells evenly weighted in each hand.

INCLINE BENCH FLYES

As with the flat dumbbell press, this exercise can be performed with a flat or inclined bench. If you are inclining the bench, assume the start position as for the flat bench flyes. Lift the dumbbells in an arc above your chest until your knuckles almost touch, exhaling as you do so. Lower the weights through the same range, inhaling. Only lower to a position of mild stretch.

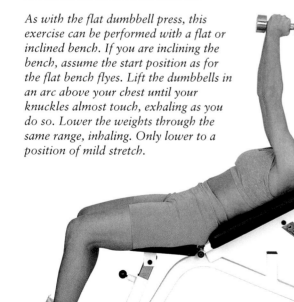

FLAT BENCH FLYES:

Works the pectorals, front deltoids

Keep the abdominals contracted and lower your back flat onto a bench or step. Assume the starting position as shown with arms open wide but with elbows soft. Follow the same procedure as for the incline bench flyes.

PEC DEC: *Works pectorals, front deltoids*

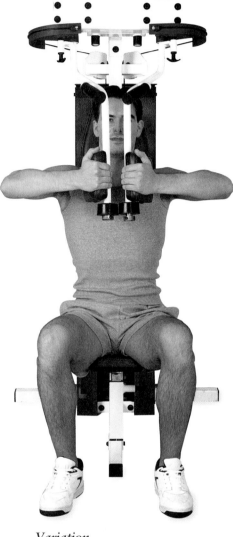

This machine can be adjusted to increase or reduce the weight you are working with, so check the weight stack before you begin and adjust for your preferred intensity. The height of the seat can also be altered to ensure your shoulders and arms are working at the correct angle – approximately 90°. As a beginner you should perform one set of 10–20 repetitions for the first four weeks, building up to three sets by week 9.

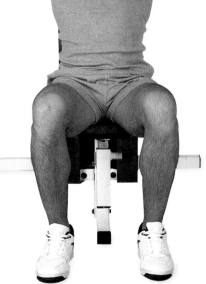

1 *Start with a light, overhand grip. Keep your back straight against the support, your chest lifted and your abdominals contracted. Keep your feet flat on the floor. Place your forearms flat against the pads, with your hands relaxed. Breathe in.*

Variation

This variation will make the pec dec easier for people with shoulder problems. Grip the elbow pads with an inward grip. Perform the exercise as for steps 1 and 2 above but make sure the elbows do not lock out.

2 *Exhaling, squeeze the pads together in a controlled movement to finish in front of your face. Inhaling, slowly return the pads to the starting position. Timing: 4 seconds in, 4 seconds back.*

The Back

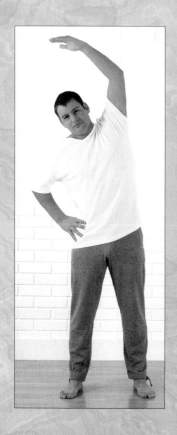

A strong back is vital for almost every activity we perform, from lifting and carrying to walking, and yet back pain is one of the most common complaints people experience. Regular back strengthening exercises can do much to alleviate aches.

A strong, flexible back is essential for your strength and mobility. Every movement of your body is dependent on the health of the muscles of your back and even the slightest injury or weakness can lead to incapacitating pain. It makes sense, therefore, for everyone to make regular stretching and toning of the muscles of the back an integral feature of an exercise programme.

The anatomy of the back

The trapezius is the largest of the back muscles. It is roughly diamond-shaped and extends from the base of the skull to the lowest thoracic vertebrae and across the full width of the back, where it is attached to both shoulder blades and collarbones. It is usually divided up into the upper, middle and lower trapezius. The way in which the trapezius is attached enables it to perform many different actions. The upper trapezius helps to support the head and neck, shrugs the shoulders and stabilises the shoulders when carrying heavy loads. The middle and lower trapezius stabilise the shoulder blades and retract or 'brace' the shoulders during arm movements.

The rhomboid muscles are connected to the upper vertebrae and

COMPLEMENTARY BACK EXERCISE

▶ Swimming is excellent for developing strong back muscles.

▶ Rowing is not only one of the best general forms of exercise you can perform, it also specifically strengthens the back.

▶ Most forms of gardening, including digging, using a fork, or lifting a wheelbarrow strengthen the back, although good posture is vital.

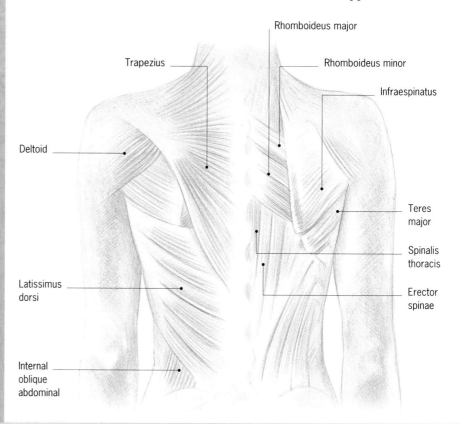

the shoulder blades and work with the middle and lower trapezius. Their function is to brace the shoulder blades.

The two latissimus dorsi are powerful, triangular muscles found on either side of the lower back. One side of each muscle is connected to the pelvis and the lower thoracic vertebrae while the other is attached to the back of the upper arm via a strong tendon. Each muscle moves an upper arm through a wide range of movements. Its main action involves pulling the raised arm down to the side of the body (adduction) against resistance. Acting in reverse, with the arm fixed, it pulls the trunk towards the arm, as when performing 'chin-ups'.

Back problems

Two common back problems are upper and lower crossed syndromes, which put stress on the vertebrae and intervertebral discs. In upper crossed syndrome, the pectoral and upper trapezius muscles are tight, while the rhomboids and deep neck flexors are weak. In lower crossed syndrome the hip flexors and lower back extensors tighten while the abdominals and buttocks (gluteals) weaken. In both syndromes bad posture and often pain result. This muscular stress also alters the muscles' normal mechanics and can cause irreversible damage. Where the vertebrae rub together, degeneration may occur, leading to osteoarthritis.

Altered vertebral alignment in the lower back can also place uneven stress on the intervertebral discs. With repeated wear-and-tear, the discs may rupture (prolapse), placing pressure on the nerve roots leading to sciatica, in which a sharp pain is experienced in the leg.

Regular exercise, but also paying proper attention to posture and alignment, is vital for the health of your back. The Alexander technique may help with longstanding posture problems.

SHAPE CHALLENGE
Lower crossed syndrome

People with a poor sitting posture can develop the condition called lower crossed syndrome. It is one of the most common causes of lower back pain. As the lumbar spine is pulled forwards, the intervertebral discs are compressed and the vertebrae rub together, causing pain.

Because so many occupations are now primarily sedentary this problem is becoming increasingly widespread, but exercise can bring about major improvements.

CASE HISTORY
Mary is a 48-year-old receptionist in a government housing agency. Most of her day is spent at her desk, answering the phone, greeting visitors, or typing. Over the last few months she has developed lower back pain. Her doctor has recommended she take regular breaks to stretch her back throughout the working day, but because her desk must always be manned, Mary finds it virtually impossible to do so.

Mary's regime
▶ *It is essential that Mary start stretching her hip flexors and low back extensors every morning and evening to restore them to a normal length. The abdominals can then be strengthened with crunches and the gluteals with lunges. It is also important to develop endurance in the low back extensors using exercises such as 'superman'.*

▶ *Mary should also improve her seated posture with the advice of an Alexander technique therapist. Sitting with her spine straight and shoulders back will be beneficial.*

SHAPE CHALLENGE
Upper crossed syndrome

Incorrect training in which the chest muscles are overworked while little attention is paid to the upper back, can lead to a common pattern of muscular imbalances called upper crossed syndrome. This condition is often seen simply as a case of 'poor posture' – chin poking forwards and rounded shoulders. It may lead to shoulder and neck pain or injury during many normal movements, and so the problem is important to address.

CASE HISTORY
Michael is a 45-year-old self-employed plumber. Having become recently concerned about his expanding waistline and sagging pectorals, Michael joined his local gym. He has concentrated on working his chest muscles in order to improve his chest shape. Although he's been attending the gym for two months, and has also made changes to his diet, he's been disappointed to find his stomach still looks larger than his chest.

Michael's regime
▶ *Michael needs to redirect his training towards the muscles of the upper back to balance his physique. He must begin by regularly stretching the upper trapezius and pectorals until they reach their desirable length. To help to return the shoulders to a neutral position, his weakened rhomboids should be trained with exercises such as the seated row, single arm dumbbell rows or reverse flyes.*

▶ *He should also examine his posture for signs of weakness, as this could be affecting his shape.*

Exercises to target the back

Stretching the back is absolutely vital before beginning any form of exercise. If you fail to stretch properly you could easily strain a muscle causing pain and even immobility. It is also important to have a comfortable exercise mat to work on to avoid pressing on sensitive spinal nerves. Mats are readily available in most sports stores.

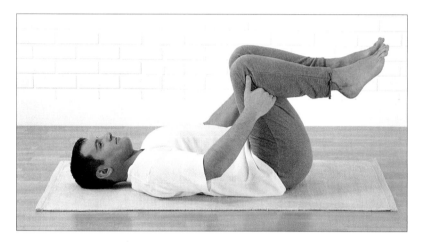

BACK STRETCHES

Lower back stretch

Lie on your back. Grip your legs underneath your knees at the back of your thighs and ease the legs in towards the body. Keep your body aligned and ensure that your head and neck remain relaxed. Hold the stretch for 10–20 seconds and breathe easily throughout. As a variation to this stretch, rest your lower legs on a chair with hips and knees at 90° to body.

Lower back rotation stretch

1 *Lie on your back with your whole body aligned. Stretch your arms out at shoulder height, 90° to your body. Bend one leg.*

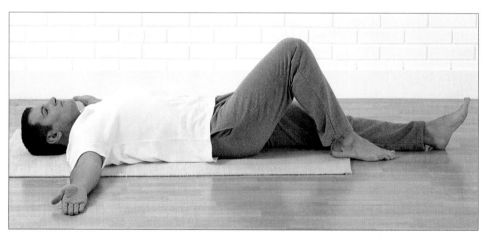

2 *Bring the knee across the mid-line of the body, allowing it to slowly fall to the opposite side: stop when you feel a comfortable stretch. If desired, place your hand on your outer thigh and apply gentle pressure to ease the stretch further. Hold the stretch 10–20 seconds, then relax, return to the starting position and repeat on the other side. As a variation you can perform this stretch by bending both knees together. Then slowly ease both knees down to the floor, first towards your left side, and then towards your right.*

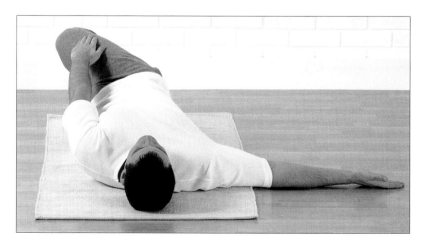

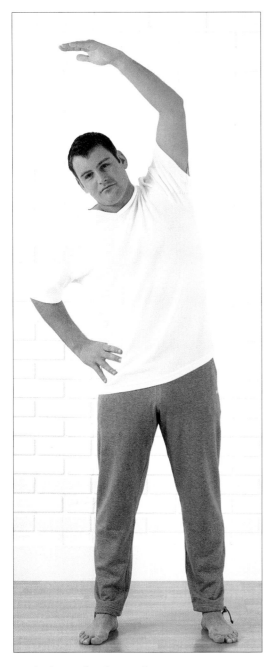

Latissimus dorsi stretch

Stand with feet hip-width apart and your abdominals contracted. Hold one arm straight overhead. Lean sideways from the hip joint but keep the hips level. Extend your arm until a stretch is felt. Hold the stretch for 10–20 seconds, breathing easily throughout. Repeat the stretch on the other side.

SEATED ROW: *Works the rhomboids, latissimus dorsi*

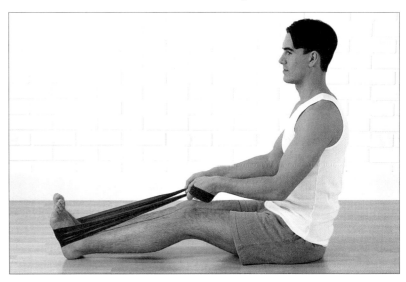

1 *An elastic band is needed for this exercise. Sit on the floor with legs extended in front of you (bend your knees slightly to make easier). Make sure that your back is straight and abdominals contracted. Pull the elastic with your arms until there is a slight tension in the elastic band.*

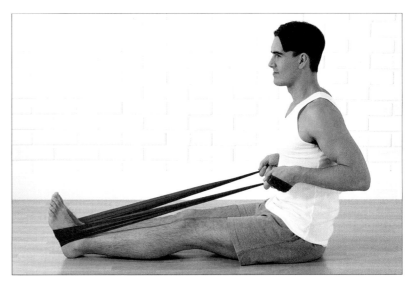

2 *Squeeze your elbows slowly backwards increasing the tension in the elastic band. Exhale as you do this. Inhale as you return slowly to step 1. Keep your back straight and your abdominals contracted throughout.*

Don't lean back too far and allow your back to arch. This places stress on your lower back.

Don't lift your shoulders up towards your ears; this may produce pain in the neck.

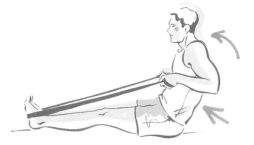

SINGLE ARM DUMBBELL ROW: *Works rhomboids, latissimus dorsi*

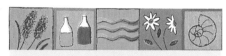

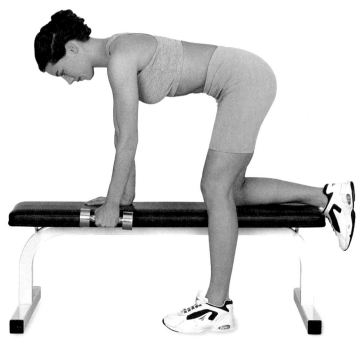

1 *For this exercise you will need a bench or step and a dumbbell. Support your body weight equally with one leg and arm on the bench, as shown.*

It is important to keep a slight bend in the leg that is standing. Keep your abdominals contracted and your back horizontal.

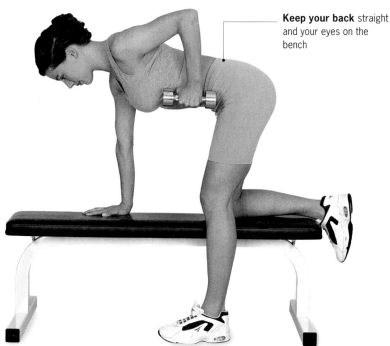

Keep your back straight and your eyes on the bench

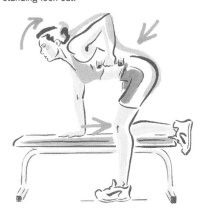

Don't lift your head up. This places stress on the back of the neck and may cause injury.

Don't let the abdominals sag. This places strain on the lower back.

Don't let the knee of the leg that is standing lock out.

2 *Lift the dumbbell upwards, keeping your elbow close to your side and breathe out. Slowly return to start position, inhaling. Your speed of*

movement should be 4 seconds up and 4 seconds down. Repeat the exercise up to ten times before switching sides to exercise the other arm.

SUPERMAN: *Works upper and lower back extensors, gluteals*

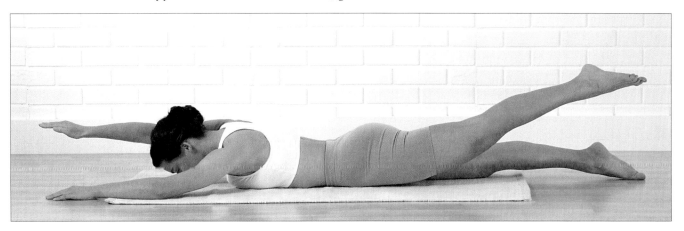

Lie on your front with your whole body in line and with a slight bend in your elbows and knees. Keep your head and neck relaxed. Lift opposite arm and leg together in a slow, controlled movement, *raising your leg to a comfortable height. Hold briefly and squeeze the muscle. Breathe out. Lower your leg slowly and with control, inhaling as you finish. Repeat with the other arm and leg.*

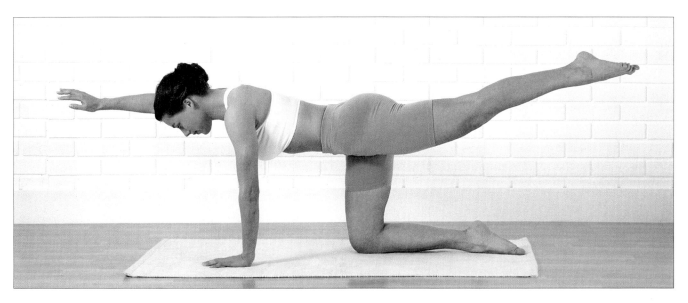

Advanced position

To increase the intensity of the superman exercise, come up onto all fours with knees hip-width apart and hands at shoulder width. Keep elbows unlocked, *spine straight and eyes facing down. Slowly raise right arm and left leg until horizontal. Keep knees and elbows unlocked. Squeeze briefly at the top position. Repeat with other arm and leg.*

Don't allow your hip to rise from the mat as this places the lower back in a strained, twisted position.

Don't allow your neck to crane backwards as this strains the spine and neck.

Don't allow your knee to bend excessively. Move smoothly to 'up' position – don't jerk.

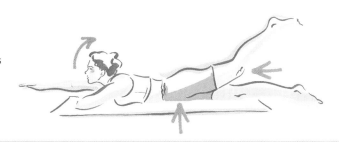

LATERAL PULL DOWN: *Works the latissimus dorsi*

Before beginning this exercise check the weight load in the pin stack, and adjust the seat level to your height. This machine also develops strength in the back of the arms, specifically the biceps.

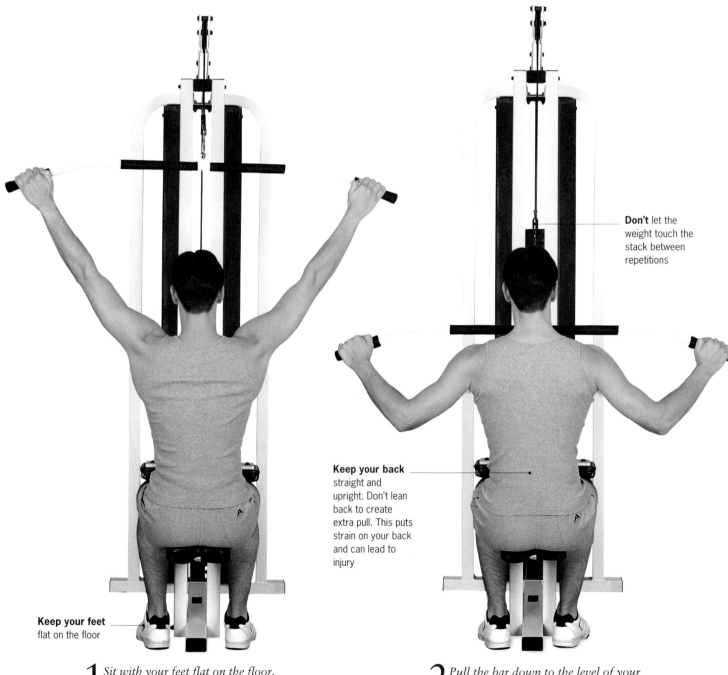

Don't let the weight touch the stack between repetitions

Keep your back straight and upright. Don't lean back to create extra pull. This puts strain on your back and can lead to injury

Keep your feet flat on the floor

1 *Sit with your feet flat on the floor, abdominals contracted and your back straight. Your lower body is stabilised by the leg pad which rests on your thighs. Use a wide overhand grip.*

2 *Pull the bar down to the level of your upper chest, exhaling. Squeeze your back muscles at the bottom position. Slowly return the bar to the start position, inhaling. Timing: 4 seconds down, 4 seconds up. Start with one set of 10–20 repetitions of the exercise in the first four weeks, building up to three sets by week 9.*

REVERSE FLYES:

*Works rhomboids,
deltoids, latissimus
dorsi, biceps*

1 *Sit with your feet
together. Keep the
abdominals contracted
and back flat. Lean
forwards. Begin with
the dumbbells down
underneath your legs.
Keep your elbows
slightly bent.*

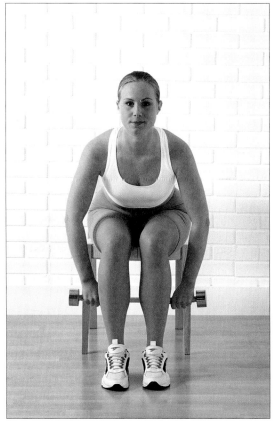

2 *Squeeze your elbows
upwards and
backwards until they
are parallel to your
body at shoulder height.
Hold at the top position
and return to starting
position in a slow,
controlled movement.
Keep your neck relaxed
throughout.*

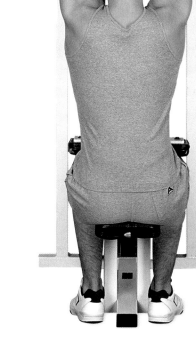

Variation
*If you have shoulder problems you will
find this variation on the pull down easier.
Grip the bar with your palms backwards
and pull it down until it is level with the
upper chest. Squeeze your back muscles at
bottom position. Return the bar to start
position in a controlled movement.*

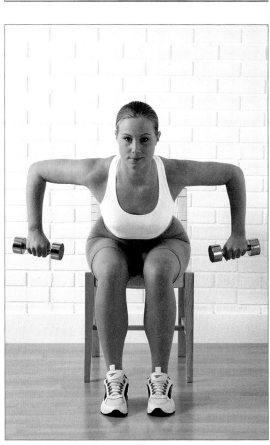

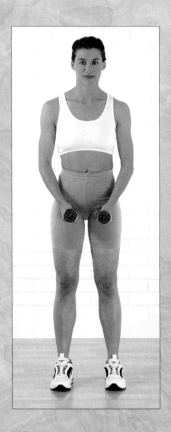

Arms and Hands

Strength in the arms and hands is essential for a wide range of daily activities, from being able to perform everyday chores to enjoying your favourite leisure pursuits. It is relatively easy to target the relevant muscles to achieve rapid improvements.

Both men and women can lose muscle tone, particularly in the biceps, quite quickly. Any extended period of resting your muscles will cause them to waste to a degree. This will affect both your appearance and the ease with which you perform daily chores.

The anatomy of the arm

The main muscles of the upper arms are the deltoid, biceps and triceps. Although these muscles have individual actions, they are often used as assistors to the larger chest and back muscles during normal activities.

The deltoid is a V-shaped muscle, originating from the collar bone (clavicle) and the top of the shoulder blade (scapula) and connected to the side of the upper arm. It is divided into three parts: the front, middle and rear deltoid, each with distinct actions. The middle deltoid is the most powerful of the three, and is mainly responsible for raising the arm from the side of the body (abduction). The front deltoid assists the upper pectoral in lifting the arm in front of the body. Working in conjunction with the rhomboids, the rear deltoid pulls the arm backwards from in front of the body.

COMPLEMENTARY ARMS AND HANDS EXERCISE

▶ Climbing is an excellent sport for developing both arm and hand strength. You don't have to climb outdoors; indoor climbing centres are becoming increasingly popular, and are an excellent and safe way to develop your expertise.

▶ Martial arts place great emphasis on arm strength and flexibility. Judo, karate and aikido, as well as gentler forms such as t'ai chi will all help you to build strength.

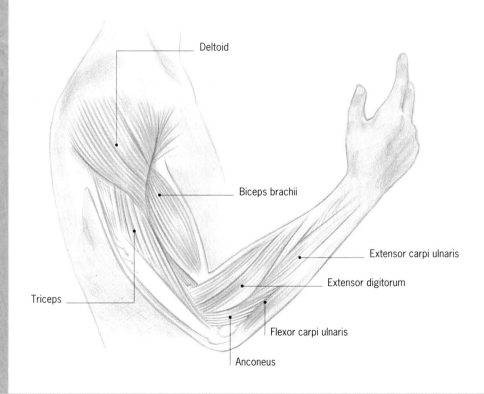

Deltoid

Biceps brachii

Extensor carpi ulnaris

Extensor digitorum

Triceps

Flexor carpi ulnaris

Anconeus

The biceps (*biceps brachii*) covers the front of the upper arm. Its main functions are to bring the forearm towards the shoulder, as when eating, or to turn the hand 'palm up', a movement called supination, as when using a screwdriver. The muscle contracts powerfully when carrying heavy weights.

The triceps covers the whole of the back of the upper arm. Its main function is to straighten the elbow joint from a bent position (extension) but only when the movement takes place against a resistance or gravity, for instance, when pushing something away from yourself. When slowly lowering the forearm, the triceps are relaxing while the biceps are contracting.

Anatomy of the hand

The muscles of the hand and fingers require precise control to carry out their numerous actions. The muscles can be broadly divided into those that bend and extend the wrist (flexors and extensors) and those which cause the hand to rotate 'palm up' or 'palm down' (supinators and pronators). Within the hand, many small muscles produce all the movements of the fingers and thumb, such as making a fist.

Arm and hand problems

A number of common muscular problems result from using muscles incorrectly. Tennis elbow is characterised by pain and tenderness on the outside of the elbow and in the back of the forearm. It is caused by inflammation of the tendon that attaches the extensor muscles to the humerus, the bone of the upper arm. Playing racquet sports with a poor grip or activities such as gardening can bring on the condition. Although rest is often recommended as treatment, addressing muscle usage is also very important.

Perhaps the most common hand problem experienced is repetitive strain injury.

SHAPE CHALLENGE
Flabby arms

In women, a major fat storage site is the back of the arms, around the triceps. The amount of fat stored here depends on overall body fat levels and on genetic and hormonal factors. If overall body fat levels are high, toning exercises alone will have little influence on arm shape (remember that muscles lie underneath the visible body fat). Body fat must be reduced with a programme of diet and aerobic exercise, together with toning work.

CASE HISTORY

Dorothy is 55 years old, and has recently retired from work as a nursing auxiliary. While her job was quite demanding physically, involving some heavy lifting and cleaning duties, now that she has retired Dorothy has felt entitled to a break and has been quite inactive. After a few weeks' relaxation she decided to rejoin her local bowling club. She was shocked to discover she quickly felt tired with severe aches and pains, and had very little upper arm strength.

Dorothy's regime

▶ *Dorothy has quickly lost the upper arm strength she developed while nursing . She must recognise that now that she is retired she will need some specific form of exercise to maintain muscle strength. Bowling will be a useful sport in the long term, but initially she needs to rebuild strength by performing specific exercises such as the dumbbell lateral raise and the triceps dip. She may also need to reassess her diet to cut back on excess fat.*

SHAPE CHALLENGE
Repetitive strain

Although mainly associated with keyboard operators and assembly line workers, repetitive strain injury can affect anyone who repeatedly uses particular muscles in their occupation. Musicians are commonly affected, the thumb and fingers being a source of problems for players of woodwind instruments. Symptoms include pain and stiffness in the affected joint. Although rest is recommended to ease the problem, this is often impractical for long periods.

CASE HISTORY

Robert is 40 years old and a member of a jazz group in which he plays the flute. The group members are thrilled that their bookings have recently increased dramatically, and from being a part-time hobby, the group now appears on the verge of being commercially successful. Robert has given up his part-time job in a local library to concentrate on his music, but is distressed to find that his playing has become severely hampered by stiffness and pain in his fingers.

Robert's regime

▶ *Robert's hands did not have sufficient time to adjust to the new demands placed on them. He needs to introduce a regular programme of stretching to warm and loosen his muscles before he begins practising each day. Squeezing a tennis ball daily may help develop muscle strength in the other muscles of the fingers.*

▶ *Robert also needs to take some breaks from his music. A hobby such as t'ai chi will be relaxing and may ease his muscle strain.*

Exercises to target the arms

Even if you think you regularly exercise the muscles of your arms through daily activities, specific exercises using weights can help you to target areas of weakness. After a few weeks of strengthening exercises you should notice a rapid improvement in your ability to carry shopping, perform household chores, even help yourself out of the bath.

ARM STRETCHES

Triceps stretch

This stretch can be performed in a sitting or standing position. With your abdominals contracted and your back straight, place the fingers of one hand between your shoulder blades. Support this arm with the other other hand as shown. Apply pressure towards the back of the head, and push the elbow down your spine with the supporting hand. Feel the stretch in the back of the arm. Breathe evenly throughout and repeat for the other side.

If this stretch is uncomfortable, take the support arm in front of the head and push the arm from lower down.

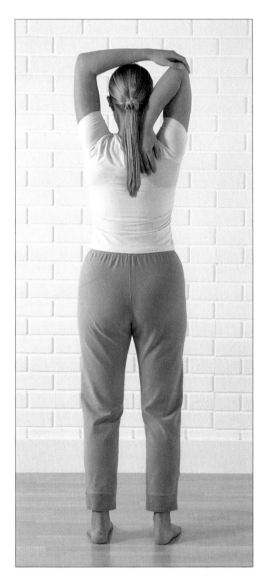

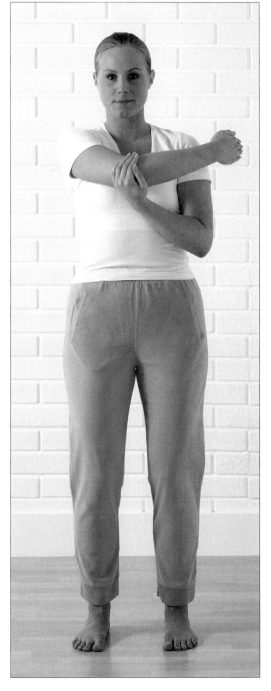

Shoulder stretch ▶

Stand with feet hip-width apart, abdominals contracted and knees unlocked. Bring one arm across the front of the body at shoulder height. Support the arm at the elbow with the other hand and ease the arm farther across the body until the stretch is felt in the shoulder.

BICEPS CURL

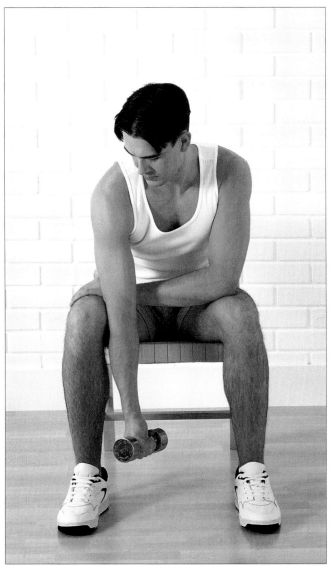

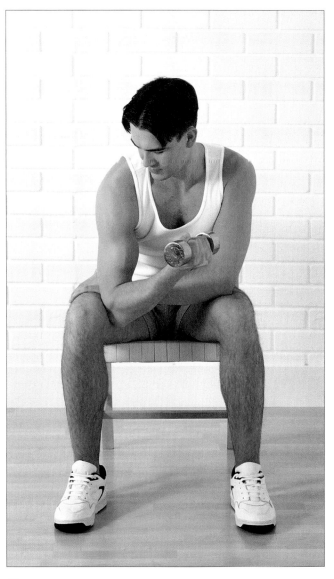

1 *Sit on a bench or chair with feet just wider than hip-width apart. With your abdominals contracted, lean slightly forwards with your back straight. Slowly straighten the arm carrying the dumbbell towards the floor, keeping it supported at the elbow by the other arm and the inner thigh.*

2 *Moving only the exercising arm, squeeze the dumbbell upwards until level with your shoulder, exhaling as you do so. Momentarily squeeze your bicep at the top position. In a slow, controlled movement, lower your arm to start position.*

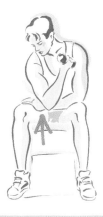

Don't allow your elbow to lift away from the contact with your inner thigh and supporting arm. This makes the exercise much less effective.

DUMBBELL LATERAL RAISE: *Works the deltoids*

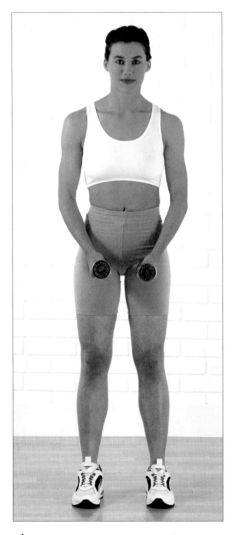

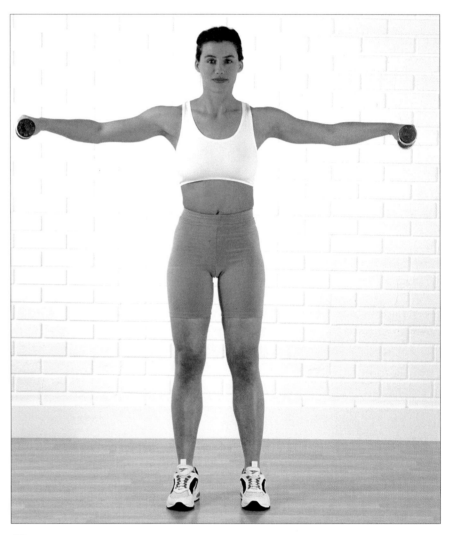

1 *Stand with abdominals contracted, back straight and knees slightly bent. Start with the dumbbells lowered together in front of your body and a small bend in the elbows.*

2 *Lift the dumbbells sideways away from your body until your arms are level with your shoulders, exhaling as you do so. In a slow and controlled*

movement, lower the weights to the start position, inhaling. If possible, perform this exercise in front of a mirror to check your technique and body symmetry.

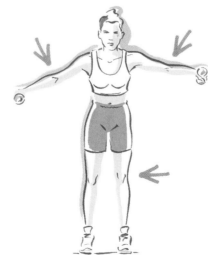

Don't lean forwards with knees locked as this can put excessive strain on the lower back. Arms should be level: use a mirror to check correct arm height and symmetry.

Don't allow elbows to lock out as this can strain the elbow joint.

SHOULDER PRESS: *Works the deltoids and triceps*

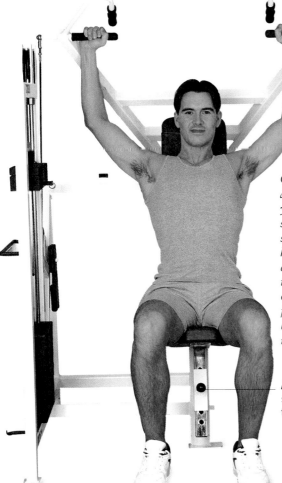

Remember to check the weight stack and adjust the seat. Sit with your feet flat on the floor. Grip the bars so your palms are facing the front. Keep your back against the back support pad. Exhaling, slowly pull down until your hands are level with your ears. Inhaling, slowly return to start position. Start with one set of 10–20 repetitions for the first four weeks, building to three sets by week 9.

Adjust the seat
so that the angle of
the knee bend is 90°

SANDALWOOD

Sandalwood is a very useful essential oil for soothing irritated and inflamed skin conditions. It has been valued as a cosmetic from the earliest times, and was a very important spice traded by the Dutch East India Company.

Regular exercise can lead to rough, hard or irritated skin, which sandalwood-based lotions and creams can help to heal. Recent evidence suggests that sandalwood helps to increase surface skin cell turnover, leading to a fresher complexion.

MACHINE TRICEPS DIP

Grip the handles with an overhand grip. Exhaling, push the handles in a slow controlled movement until they are level with the seat of the machine. Inhaling, slowly return to start position. Start with one set of 10–20 repetitions for the first four weeks building to three sets by week 9.

If rollers are present, place
your legs in front of the first
and behind the second – they
serve to keep your legs still

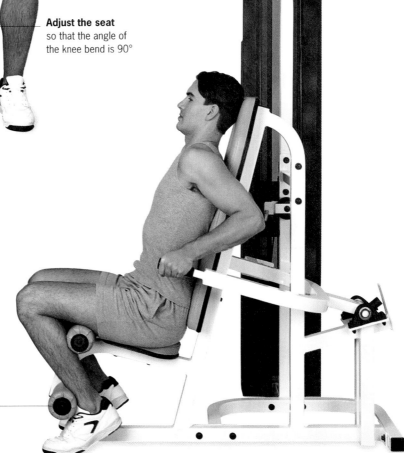

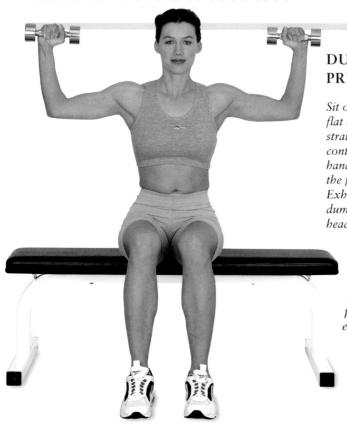

DUMBBELL SHOULDER PRESS: *Works the deltoids*

Sit on a bench with feet flat on the floor, back straight and abdominals contracted. Turn your hands so the palms face the front to start. Exhaling, raise the dumbbells above your head, keeping a bend in the elbows. Inhaling, bring your arms down to the starting position, with your elbows at 90°.

Don't 'sit' on your toes. This is an unstable position and can lead to injury.

Don't allow the dumbbells to fall back over the head. This causes the lower back to arch and can result in injury.

MACHINE BICEPS CURL

Keep your feet flat on the floor and back straight. Grasp the handles with an underhand grip. Arms should be almost straight and elbows unlocked. Contracting the biceps muscle, curl the bar towards you, exhaling. Squeeze biceps at end of movement (as shown) and return to start position.

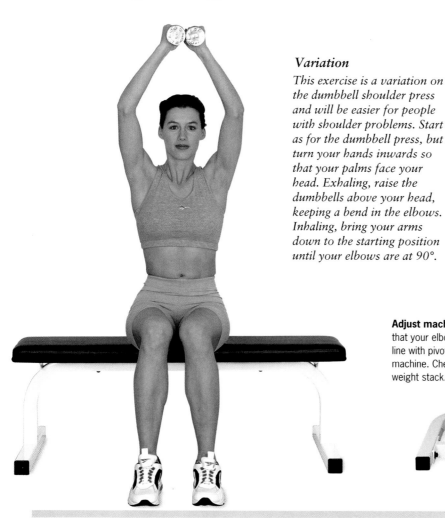

Variation

This exercise is a variation on the dumbbell shoulder press and will be easier for people with shoulder problems. Start as for the dumbbell press, but turn your hands inwards so that your palms face your head. Exhaling, raise the dumbbells above your head, keeping a bend in the elbows. Inhaling, bring your arms down to the starting position until your elbows are at 90°.

Adjust machine so that your elbow is in line with pivot of machine. Check the weight stack.

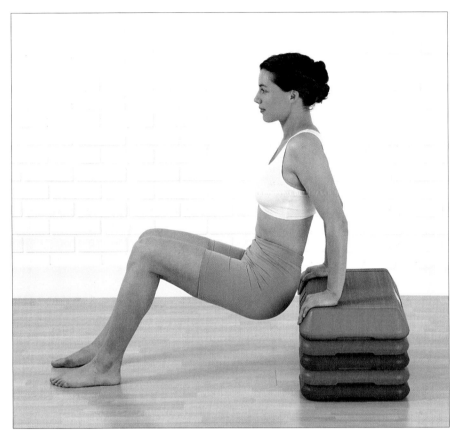

TRICEPS DIP

1 *Place your hands facing forwards on a step or bench, shoulder-width apart so that your arms take your body weight. Keep a bend in your knees and place your feet shoulder-width apart, flat on the floor. It is important to ensure the step or bench is at the correct height. If the step is too low the exercise will not be effective as you will not be fully extending the triceps muscle. If the step is too high your body will be at too extreme an angle.*

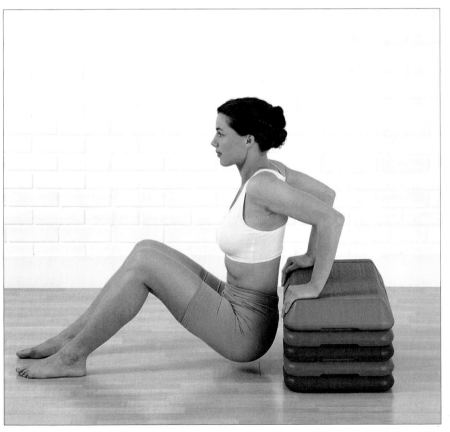

2 *Inhaling, slowly lower your body by bending the elbows – do not bend them beyond 90°. If you experience shoulder pain, only bend to a comfortable position. Keep your bottom close to the step or bench at all times. Push upwards to the start position and exhale. Your elbows should remain slightly bent at the top position.*

Don't place your feet too far away from the step. This will cause the body to lower at an angle and place undue strain on the shoulder joints.

Don't lock out the elbows on the up phase of the exercise – maintain a slight bend. On the down phase of the exercise, the arms should be lowered to 90° at the elbow joint.

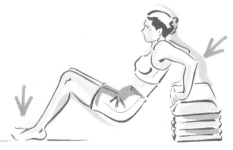

Exercises to target the hands

You may imagine your hands get sufficient exercise from daily activities so that specific strengthening exercises are unnecessary. However, when you consider how important your hands are to every aspect of your life, and when the incidence of problems such as repetitive strain injury is on the increase, it makes good sense to give your hands a daily work-out. Most of these exercises can easily be performed at a desk or even while watching television.

WRIST EXERCISES: *Works the extensors, flexors*

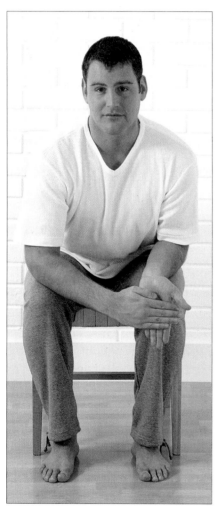

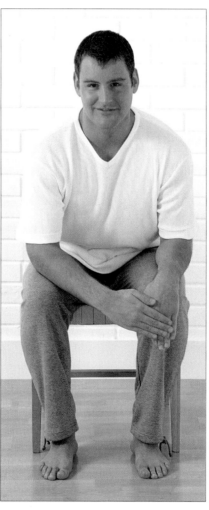

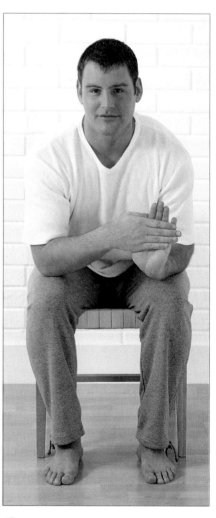

1 *Sit on a chair with your left hand hanging over the edge of your left knee, palm upwards. Ensure the lower arm is in contact with your thigh at all times. Follow the sequence holding each stretch for 10–30 seconds. Start with a flexor stretch: using your right hand to control the movement of the left, bend your hand down until you can feel an easy stretch in the back of the forearm.*

2 *Moving to an extensor stretch, turn your palm so that it faces downwards. Apply downward pressure until you can feel an easy stretch in the wrist and forearm.*

3 *From this 'down' position gently ease the hand backwards until you can feel the stretch. Repeat the sequence with the other hand.*

WRIST MOBILITY EXERCISES

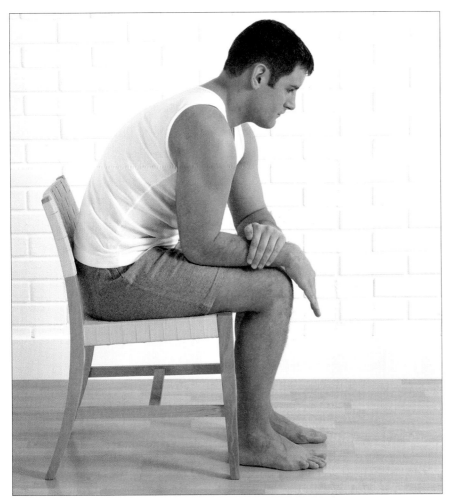

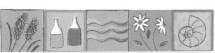

LAVENDER OIL

Lavender oil is one of the most important of the essential oils. It can rapidly heal scar tissue and so is ideal for cuts and burns. Its properties were first discovered accidentally by the developer of aromatherapy, René Gattefosse, who found it healed a bad burn quickly and without scarring. Lavender oil is suitable for most skin types except very dry, sensitive skin. To make a healing cuticle cream, add 5 drops of lavender oil and 10 drops of tea tree oil to a base cream.

1 *Sit on a chair with your right hand hanging over the edge of your right knee, palm facing downwards and supported at the wrist by your left hand. Follow the sequence slowly and hold each position for two seconds. Repeat the cycle four times, then change to the other hand. To increase the intensity, hold a light weight in the hand.*

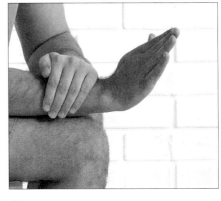

2 *From the 'down' position, ease the hand up as far as it will go so that you feel a gentle stretch. Then turn the hand so that the thumb points upwards.*

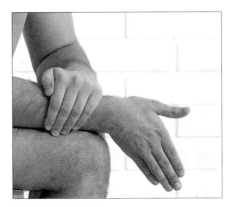

3 *Now bend the hand down again, keeping the wrist joint supported on the thigh with the other hand.*

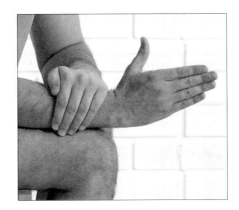

4 *Gently ease the hand up again as far as it will go until an easy stretch is felt. Slowly return to start position.*

The Abdomen

In most people the abdominal muscles are relatively weak and overstretched. They usually require strengthening rather than stretching. Toning this area will not only improve your shape, but also help your posture, and may even relieve back pain.

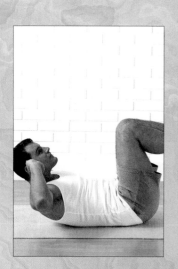

COMPLEMENTARY ABDOMEN EXERCISE

▶ It is essential to build good abdominal tone before performing vigorous activities; if your trunk is unstable you could injure yourself. However, once basic tone is established, exercises such as tennis, golf, yoga and t'ai chi are excellent for maintaining or improving abdominal tone.

▶ When performed with correct technique, lifting and carrying, gardening or weight training provide a good abdominal work-out.

The abdomen is one of the most common problem areas of the body. As a major site of fat storage for both men and women it is the area where you will probably first notice any weight gain, yet it is often quite difficult to isolate and target the stomach muscles when exercising. For example, exercises such as full sit-ups only use the abdominal muscles for the first 30 degrees of the movement: after that the hip flexors complete the motion. These exercises can also lead to injury as the hip flexors pull on the spine, altering posture and increasing disc pressure. Any exercises which extend the muscles from a prone position may be unsuitable for people with back conditions such as a prolapsed disc or a history of lower back pain. In these cases you should consult your doctor before attempting them.

For women, pregnancy places particular demands on the muscles of the abdomen and returning them to their former strength can be a challenge.

The anatomy of the abdomen
There are four main abdominal muscles – the rectus abdominis, the internal and external obliques, and the transversus abdominis. They provide stability for the trunk and

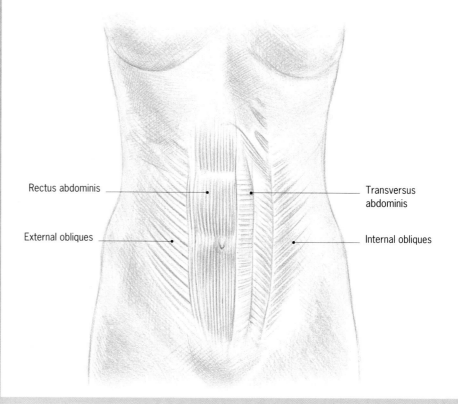

Rectus abdominis

Transversus abdominis

External obliques

Internal obliques

protect and support the digestive organs. Many abdominal exercises use all four muscles, although their individual actions can be identified. The rectus abdominis flexes the trunk by pulling the lower breast bone towards the pelvis – or vice versa. The internal and external obliques work in combination to rotate the trunk. The transversus abdominis compresses the abdominal contents to flatten your abdomen and hold in your stomach.

The abdominal muscles are arranged in layers and are unusual in being joined to other muscles by their tendons; most skeletal muscles in the body are connected to bone.

Abdomen problems

After pregnancy many women find it difficult to regain the strength of their abdominal muscles. However, if correct abdominal training is performed during pregnancy, muscle tone will return more quickly following the birth. This is especially important if you intend to return to sporting activities or exercise. It is also essential to strengthen the muscles of the pelvic floor which can also be weakened after childbirth. The pelvic floor muscles act like a sling to support the pelvic organs and also help strengthen the sphincter muscle which controls the flow of urine from the bladder. Weak muscles can lead to urinary incontinence, as well as irritation of the hip and sacroiliac joints.

Another common shape problem is lordotic posture. This occurs when weak abdominal muscles fail to adequately compress the abdomen allowing it to protrude forwards. This exerts a pull on the lower spine, often leading to back pain or disc problems. Excess body fat in the area worsens the problem. Because the body tends to store more fat in the abdominal area as we age, it is particularly important to maintain abdominal tone through exercise.

SHAPE CHALLENGE
A fit pregnancy

During pregnancy the abdominal muscles stretch to allow for the baby to grow. Later on, the hormone relaxin acts on the linea alba – a tendinous sheath that joins the two sides of the rectus abdominis – causing it to soften so that it can stretch sideways thus providing more room for the baby.

Increasingly, fitness experts are finding that maintaining abdominal tone during pregnancy can help you to regain muscle strength much faster after the birth.

CASE HISTORY

Ruth is a 29-year-old woman, 20 weeks pregnant with her first child. A keen tennis player, she hopes to be able to return to playing with her club a few months after the birth. So far her pregnancy has progressed well, with little morning sickness, and Ruth has felt well enough to swim three times a week. However, as she has started to grow bigger she is feeling less confident about her exercise programme.

Ruth's regime

▶ *Ruth first needs to have a thorough check-up with her doctor and discuss her exercise plans. Her doctor will be able to advise if there are particular exercises to avoid.*

▶ *She should then visit a local gym where fitness experts will be able to advise on an exercise plan to suit her. They may suggest easier versions of crunches, oblique curls, pelvic flattening and alternating leg kicks. They may also recommend aqua-aerobics as a gentler alternative to lane swimming.*

SHAPE CHALLENGE
Lordotic posture

General weight gain combined with weak abdominal muscles can lead to the development of lordotic posture characterised by a pot-bellied appearance. This condition can also be a common cause of lower back pain. When the abdominal muscles are weak they allow the abdomen to exert a forward pull on the lower (lumbar) spine. This places stress on the vertebrae and supporting structures leading to chronic degeneration of the lumbar vertebrae and increased pressure on the vertebral discs.

CASE HISTORY

Barry is 57 years old and took early retirement last year. Although he's always been a little overweight, over the past few months he's gained a lot of weight and is embarrassed about his protruding stomach. Although he enjoys golf he's been alarmed to find himself puffed out by any exertion and has also suffered painful lower back spasms. His doctor has diagnosed lordotic posture and recommends regular exercise.

Barry's regime

▶ *Barry must develop an overall health and fitness plan in conjunction with his doctor. He must first improve his general level of fitness with some regular aerobic exercise, before turning his attention to his abdomen. It will also be essential to change his diet, cutting back on alcohol and high-fat foods.*

▶ *Once Barry's general fitness has improved he can focus on abdomen crunches and curls to strengthen his abdomen.*

Exercises to target the abdomen

The abdominals are the one group of muscles where stretching is generally not so vital. However, you should bear in mind that abdominal exercises will also work other muscles of the body such as the neck, back, legs and chest, so a thorough warm-up and general stretch is still extremely important.

PRONE EXTENSION STRETCH

Lie face down with your elbows apart and in line with your shoulders. Keep your hips and feet in contact with the floor. Breathing evenly, gently lift your breast bone off the floor and hold for 10 seconds. A stretch may be felt in the abdominals. Repeat three times.

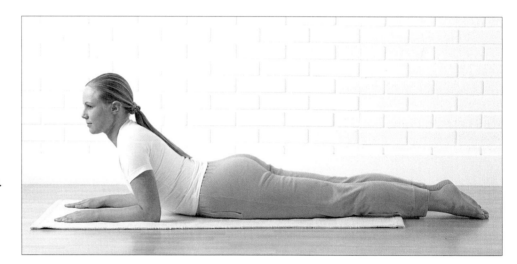

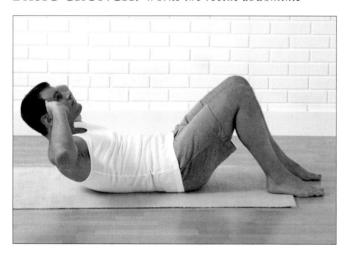

Don't perform this exercise if you have existing back problems.

Don't allow your elbows to lift off the floor. This hyperextended position places strain on the vertebrae of the lower back and may cause damage.

Don't tilt your head backwards as this places stress on the vertebrae at the back of the neck and may cause damage.

BASIC CRUNCH: *Works the rectus abdominis*

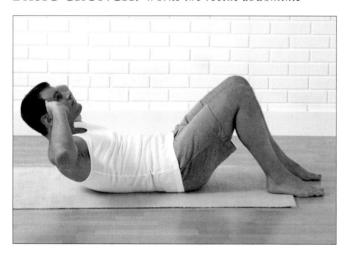

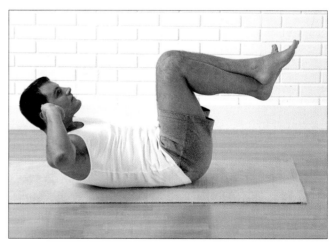

Lie on your back with your knees up, feet hip-width apart, abdominals sucked in and hands to the side of your head. Exhaling, squeeze up, raising your shoulders a little way off the floor. Hold momentarily and then slowly ease down, inhaling.

Advanced
Perform this exercise in the same way as the basic crunch, but keep both feet lifted off the floor while raising your shoulders, as shown.

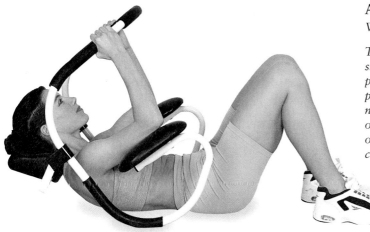

AB TRAINER CRUNCH:
Works rectus abdominis

This machine is called an ab trainer. It supports the head and neck while you perform crunches and is very useful for people who experience neck pain during normal crunches. Rest your elbows lightly on the pads and hold the frame with a light overhand grip. Keeping your lower back in contact with the floor, slowly lift your shoulders off the floor, taking the rolling frame with you.

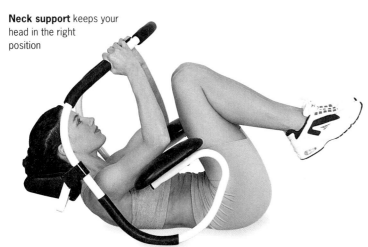

Neck support keeps your head in the right position

Advanced
Perform in the same way as the basic ab trainer crunch above, but lift up your legs at the same time as lifting your shoulders off the floor. This makes the abdominals work harder as they have to stabilise the pelvis before contracting.

Don't lift the head off the support. This makes the ab trainer less effective.

Don't pull with the arms. This makes the exercise less effective and may place stress on the neck.

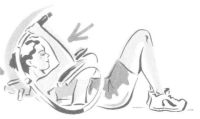

OBLIQUE CURL: *Works the internal and external obliques*

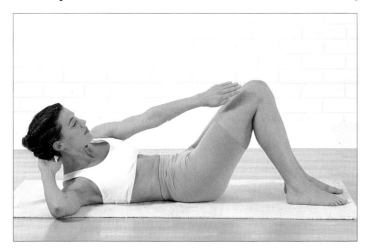

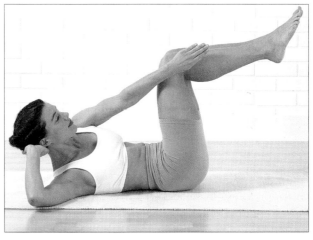

Lie flat on your back with your knees raised and feet hip-width apart. Keep your right shoulder and lower back pressed tight into floor. Exhaling, contract the abdominals and with your left arm, reach around your right knee until a stretch is felt in your mid section, while lifting your left shoulder slightly off the floor. Hold momentarily at 'top' position then, inhaling, lower back to floor.

Advanced
Perform this exercise in the same way as the oblique curl but with your knees lifted at 90° and your feet parallel. Reach up towards your toes, past your knee. As with the advanced crunch exercise this makes the oblique muscles work harder.

Legs and Feet

Healthy, strong leg and foot muscles are the basic measure of your mobility and are vital for your independence and quality of life, particularly as you age. With the increase in sedentary jobs many people are missing out an essential daily work-out.

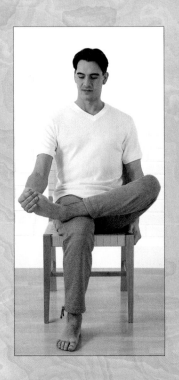

COMPLEMENTARY LEG AND FOOT EXERCISES

▶ Stair climbing is particularly good exercise for the legs and buttocks, so you don't have to use complicated machinery at the gym. Simply stepping up and down steps at home or at work for 6–12 minutes at a time will be of benefit.

▶ Ballet has always demanded a rigorous work-out for the feet, with extensive flexing and arching required. If you suffer from flat feet ballet exercises may be very beneficial.

Although a low level of fitness may first present itself as aches in the leg muscles after unaccustomed exercise, like the muscles of the arms, it is relatively easy to isolate and strengthen the muscles of the legs.

The anatomy of the legs

Covering the front of the thigh are the quadriceps. Although they consist of four separate muscles their main combined action is to straighten the knee joint (extension). The quadriceps also work during normal walking, especially down slopes or stairs where they contract to provide a breaking force. After an extensive bout of unaccustomed hill walking, it is often the quadriceps that are sore the next day.

The adductors consist of a group of muscles covering the inner thigh which bring the leg to the midline (adduction).

The main buttock muscle, gluteus maximus, is the largest muscle of the body, providing much of the power for walking upstairs or rising from a

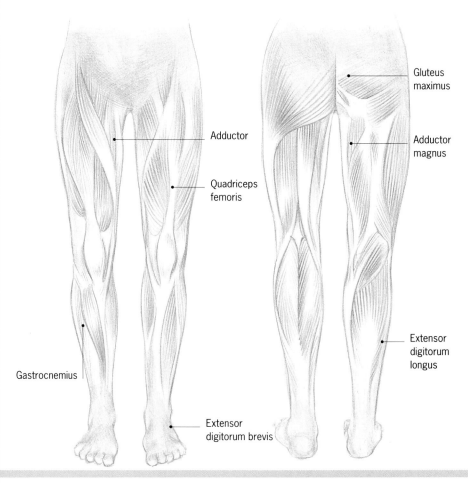

seated position. Like many of the muscles of this area, it assists with posture by maintaining the correct pelvic tilt.

The other main thigh muscles, the gluteus medius and minimus, lie underneath the gluteus maximus. They act together to lift the leg powerfully out to the side (abductors). When walking, they are extremely important in balancing the pelvis when one leg is lifted off the ground. Collectively, the gluteus muscles are known as the gluteals.

The hamstrings are at the back of the upper leg and are formed from three muscles. They cross both the hip and the knee joint and can therefore assist the gluteus maximus in pulling the leg backwards (hip extension) or work to bend the knee (flexion).

The anatomy of the feet

On the front of the lower leg is the anterior tibialis and the many extensor muscles of the toes. The anterior tibialis is the largest muscle on the front of the leg. It causes the foot to lift up (dorsiflexion). The sole of the foot consists of numerous muscles and tendons, acting to bend the toes and maintain the arch while standing or walking.

Leg and feet problems

Many women focus on their thighs as their major shape problem. In premenopausal women the thighs and buttocks are a major fat storage site, so any weight gain will see fat stored here. Toning and strengthening exercises can do much to improve appearance.

Both men and women are affected by shortening of the leg muscles, which can cause tightness and back pain. It is a common problem for people of all ages who spend long periods sitting.

Fallen arches are the most common foot shape problem, and regular exercise can help to prevent the associated pain.

SHAPE CHALLENGE
Flat feet

The arches of the feet form gradually after birth as the supportive ligaments and muscles in the soles of the feet develop. In some people arches do not form, generally because of an inherited defect, but the condition is generally painless. However, if the arches collapse in adult life the feet will generally ache when walking or standing and the toe extensors on the top of the foot can become tight and painful. Flat feet can be caused by a rapid increase in weight, or the muscles may weaken as the result of a neurological or muscular disease.

CASE HISTORY

Betty is 50 years old, and has just returned to work after recovering from a major operation. The enforced convalescence period has lead to a major weight gain, and Betty has been distressed to find walking is now very painful. Her doctor has diagnosed fallen arches and recommends she wears arch supports, but he has also advised her to undertake some exercise.

Betty's regime

▶ *Betty needs to develop with her doctor a total health and fitness programme to deal with her condition. She will need to adjust her diet and undertake some aerobic exercise to try to reduce her weight as this is contributing to the problem.*

▶ *Aerobic exercise will be difficult until her arches strengthen so she will need to perform regular arch extension exercises to build the muscles. Slowly rolling her foot over a tennis ball daily for 5 minutes will also help.*

SHAPE CHALLENGE
Tight hamstrings

Hamstrings are probably best known as the muscles which can be painfully pulled by sportsmen and women. However, the hamstrings can also be damaged more insidiously. They perform the function of bending the knee and swinging the leg backwards from the thigh. Because of this function the muscles can become shortened by long periods of sitting. The hamstrings are attached by tendons to the pelvis, so tight hamstrings will also affect the way in which the pelvis moves, and can in turn cause lower back pain.

CASE HISTORY

Jonathan is a 42-year-old executive who is largely desk-bound. Until a few months ago, he enjoyed a regular jog three times a week, but his workload has dramatically increased and he now doesn't seem to have any time for exercise. At the end of the working day Jonathan finds that he often experiences lower back ache, and that his muscles feel tight.

Jonathan's regime

▶ *Jonathan should have his back pain checked by a doctor, but it is likely that his hamstrings have shortened due to lack of activity. He must try to take regular breaks for stretching at work, 45 minutes being the maximum time he should sit without a break. He should also check his sitting posture and avoid slouching.*

▶ *Jonathan could perform some leg exercises discreetly in his chair at work. However, he also needs to make a regular time in his life for exercise once more.*

Exercises to target the legs and feet

Warming up and stretching are particularly important before beginning leg and feet exercises. Because these muscles are so vital for your general mobility, severe aches may put you off exercise altogether. This is easily avoided with proper stretching and a gradual build-up.

LEG STRETCHES

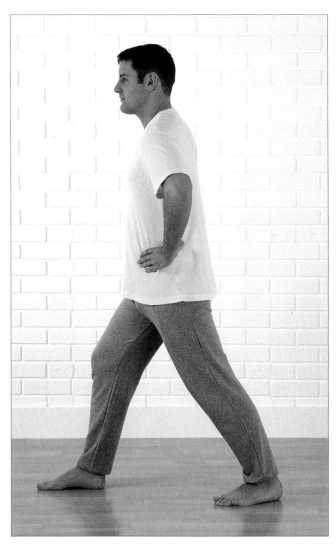

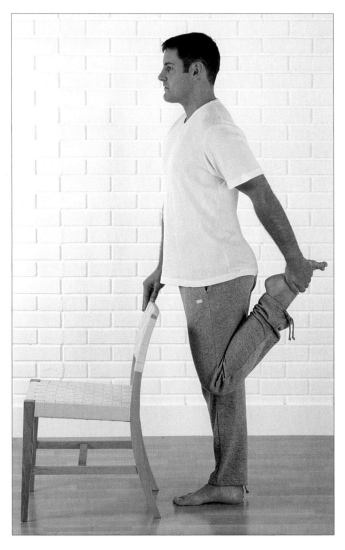

Calf stretch
Standing with your feet hip-width apart, feet facing forwards, take a step forwards with your right leg, keeping the knee slightly bent. Press the heel of the left leg into the floor until the stretch is felt in the rear calf muscle of this leg. Hold the stretch for 20–30 seconds, keeping your weight centred over your hips. Step backwards with your right leg to return to the start position. Repeat with the other leg.

Quadricep stretch
Using a chair for support, centralise your weight over your hips. Lift your left foot behind you, grasp the foot with your hand and pull it up towards your bottom, pressing the knee forwards to keep it parallel with the supporting knee. Keep the supporting knee unlocked; if possible, touch your heel to your bottom. Hold the stretch for 20–30 seconds. Lower leg slowly to the floor and repeat with the other leg.

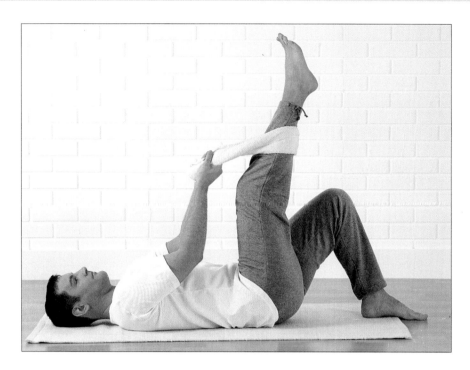

Hamstring stretch

For this stretch you will need a mat and a towel. Lie on your back with your weight evenly distributed and one knee bent. Contract the abdominals to ensure your lower back is pressed flat onto the mat. Raise your other leg and loop a towel around it. Use the towel to ease the leg gently towards the upper body until you feel a stretch. Hold the stretch for 20–30 seconds. Lower the leg slowly and repeat with the other leg.

LUNGE: *Works quadriceps, hamstrings, gluteals*

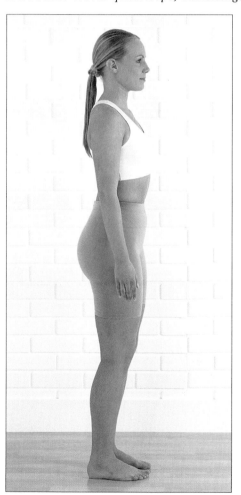

1 *Stand straight with your feet together and abdominals contracted. Throughout the exercise keep your back straight, and your head in line with your spine.*

2 *Inhaling, take a 'giant' stride with one leg, following with the body. Your front knee should not go beyond your ankle. Hold briefly at the 'bottom' position then push back to the start position, exhaling. Repeat for other leg.*

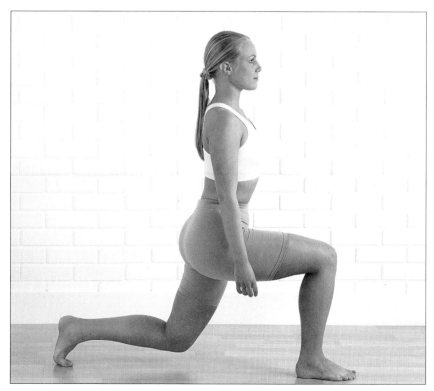

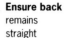

SQUAT:
Works quadriceps, hamstrings, gluteals

Stand with your abdominals contracted and feet hip-width apart. With your arms stretched out in front of you, bend at the knees, lowering the body and inhaling. Your thighs should remain above parallel to the floor and keep your head in line with your spine. Hold momentarily at 'bottom' position, then, exhaling, push up to start position.

Ensure back remains straight

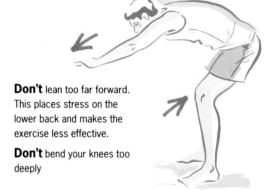

Don't lean too far forward. This places stress on the lower back and makes the exercise less effective.

Don't bend your knees too deeply

CALF RAISE

Use a chair to aid your balance. With your body straight and your abdominals contracted, press up until you are on 'tiptoes', exhaling. Momentarily hold in 'top' position before slowly lowering to the floor, inhaling.

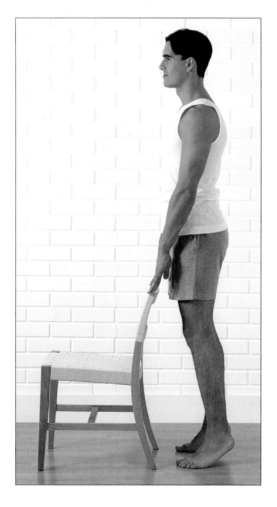

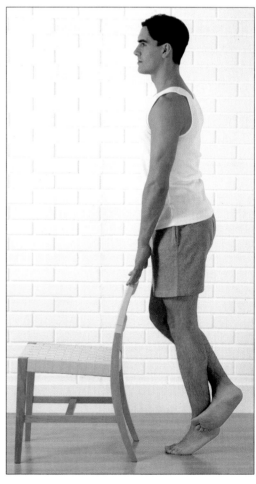

Advanced calf raise
Increase the intensity of the calf raise by performing the exercise on one foot with the other crossed behind the ankle as above.

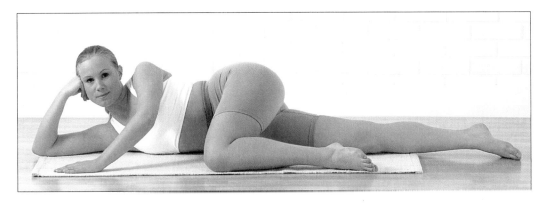

INNER THIGH RAISE:
Works adductors

1 *Lie on one side with your body aligned and one knee bent. Support your head with one hand and your body with the other as shown.*

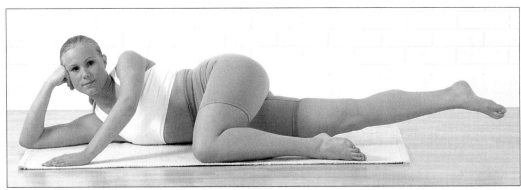

2 *With abdominals contracted and knees unlocked, slowly raise your straight leg as far as is comfortable and exhale. Keep your toes pointing down to the floor. Lower under control, and inhale. Ensure your movements are slow and controlled. Repeat with other leg.*

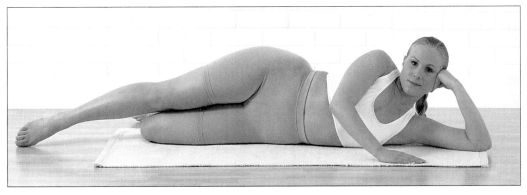

OUTER THIGH RAISE:
Works gluteals

1 *Lie on one side with the knee that is in contact with the floor bent at 90°. Support your head with one hand and your body with the other as shown.*

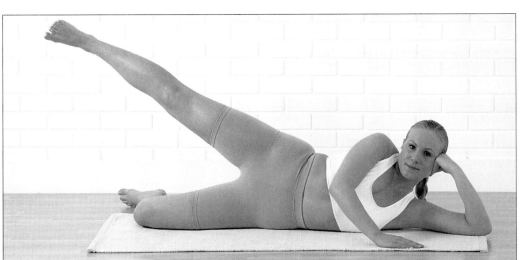

2 *With your abdominals contracted and knees unlocked, slowly raise your upper leg and exhale. Keep your toes pointing down to the floor. Lower under control, and inhale. Repeat with other leg.*

133

GLUTE LIFT:
Works gluteals

1 *You will need a mat for this exercise. Start on your hands and knees, with your hands placed directly underneath your shoulders, knees slightly apart and elbows unlocked. Looking down at the mat, contract your abdominals keeping your lower back flat. Straighten your left leg, resting on the toes of the straightened leg.*

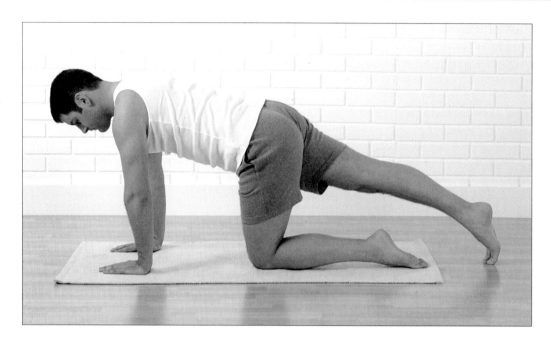

2 *Squeezing through your buttock, lift your leg to a horizontal position, concentrating on contracting the buttock. Hold the contraction for 5 seconds. Perform the exercise 10 times, then repeat with the other leg.*

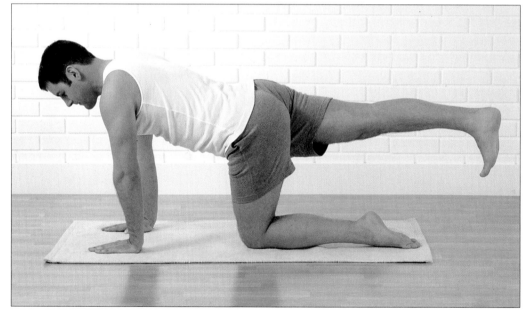

Don't tilt your head backwards as this could strain your neck.

Don't relax the abdominal muscles as your back may twist which can cause injury.

Don't allow your arms to go beyond 90° with your trunk.

Don't bend the raised leg – keep it straight with knee unlocked.

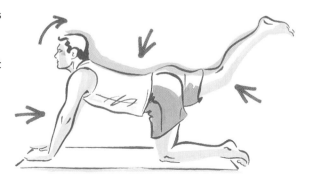

LEG PRESS:
Works quadriceps, hamstrings, gluteals

Position your feet so that the bend at your knees is 90°

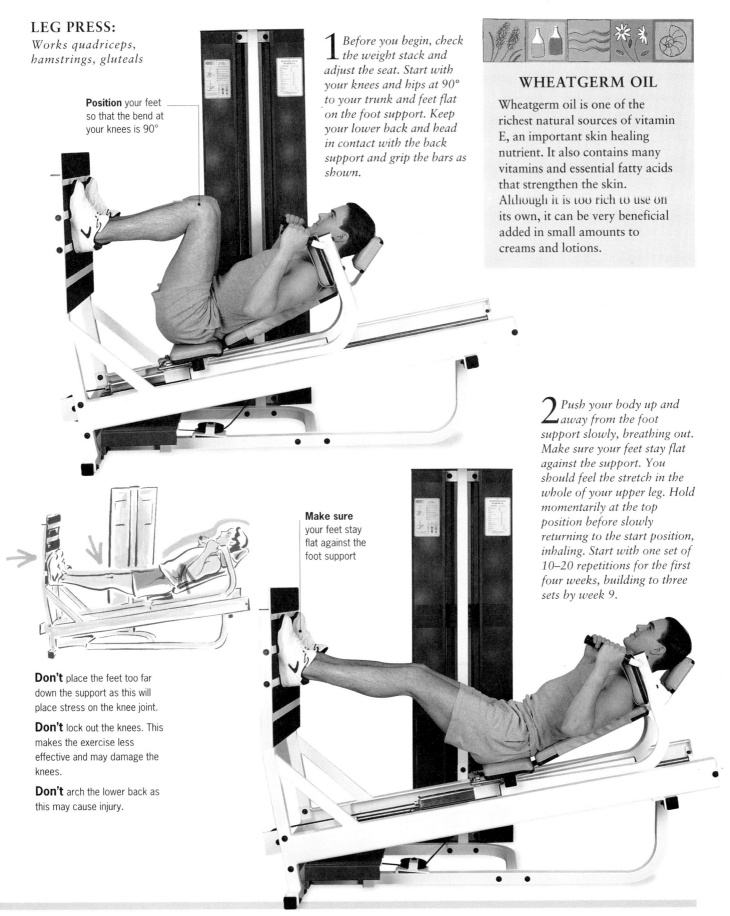

1 *Before you begin, check the weight stack and adjust the seat. Start with your knees and hips at 90° to your trunk and feet flat on the foot support. Keep your lower back and head in contact with the back support and grip the bars as shown.*

WHEATGERM OIL

Wheatgerm oil is one of the richest natural sources of vitamin E, an important skin healing nutrient. It also contains many vitamins and essential fatty acids that strengthen the skin. Although it is too rich to use on its own, it can be very beneficial added in small amounts to creams and lotions.

2 *Push your body up and away from the foot support slowly, breathing out. Make sure your feet stay flat against the support. You should feel the stretch in the whole of your upper leg. Hold momentarily at the top position before slowly returning to the start position, inhaling. Start with one set of 10–20 repetitions for the first four weeks, building to three sets by week 9.*

Make sure your feet stay flat against the foot support

Don't place the feet too far down the support as this will place stress on the knee joint.

Don't lock out the knees. This makes the exercise less effective and may damage the knees.

Don't arch the lower back as this may cause injury.

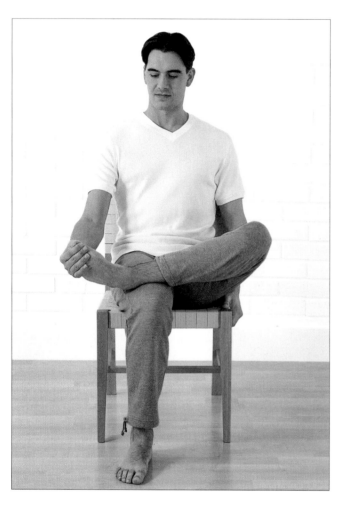

◀ TOE EXTENSORS STRETCH

Cross one leg over the other, keeping both legs in contact at all times. Grasp the foot and gently pull towards you and upwards. Hold for 10–30 seconds; repeat with the other foot.

ARCH EXERCISE

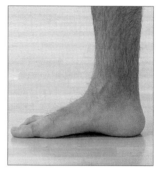

1 *This exercise will strengthen the arch of your foot and can relieve pain and tension sometimes felt as a result of fallen arches. Stand with some of your weight on one foot.*

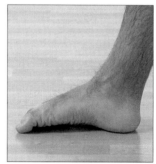

2 *Draw in your toes to arch your foot. Hold this position for 20 seconds. Now relax the foot for 20 seconds. Repeat this exercise 3–5 times with each foot.*

DORSI FLEXION: *Works anterior tibialis*

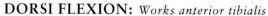

1 *You will need an elastic band. Tie the band in a loop around a fixed object, such as heavy table leg. Sit with one leg straight out in front of you. Ensure that there is mild tension in the band at this start position.*

2 *Squeeze the foot towards you. Hold at the end of the motion for 2 seconds and then slowly relax. Repeat 10–20 times.*

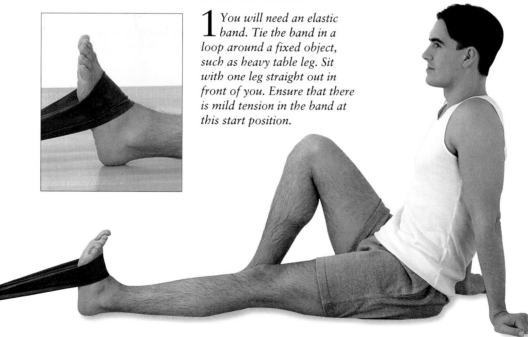

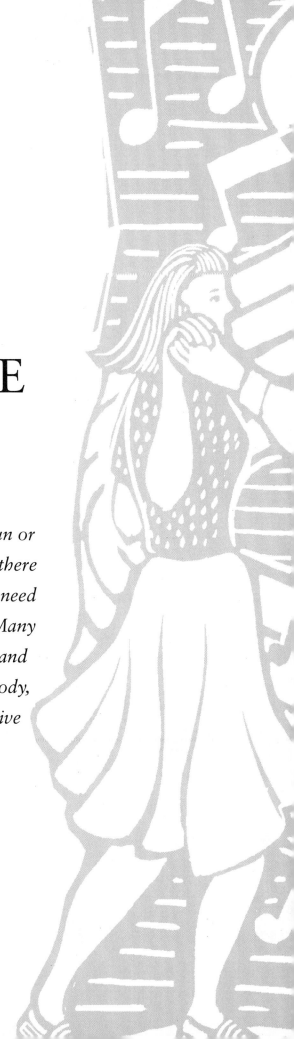

CHAPTER 6

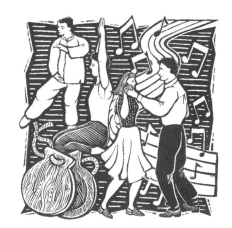

ALTERNATIVE SHAPING UP

If an action-packed aerobics class, high-impact run or a strenuous cycle ride do not appeal to you, then there are other exercise options to explore. Shaping up need never be a chore with so much choice available. Many alternative approaches focus on the mind, body and spirit as a whole, aiming not only to tone your body, but also to benefit your inner self through creative expression, meditation and relaxation.

IMPROVING BODY SHAPE WITH YOGA

The ancient Indian art of yoga is more than just a form of physical exercise. As well as improving strength and flexibility, yoga promotes inner calm and health in the internal organs.

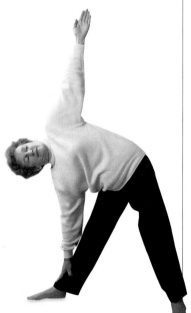

YOGA FOR FLEXIBILITY
Flexibility is one of the most important aspects of yoga. By emphasising muscle relaxation at the beginning of a routine even the most challenging positions become achievable.

Yoga has been practised in India for over 2000 years as a means of keeping both the physical body and the spiritual self healthy and working in unison with each other. It has traditionally held the unique status of being both a medicinal and spiritual therapy: used both as a practical part of Ayurvedic medicine (see page 42) and as a form of religious devotion. However, it is not necessary to subscribe to any particular set of beliefs to practise yoga; people from all cultures and walks of life can enjoy its mental and physical benefits.

From a shaping-up perspective yoga can be quite demanding and very beneficial. The various postures require both flexibility and a surprising degree of muscular strength. Stamina is also vital.

HOW YOGA WORKS

There are eight fundamental principles, or sutras, on which yoga is built. The first two are the *yamas* and *niyamas* – moral and ethical codes that help a person to conduct a life that is disciplined and does not harm any other individual. *Asana* and *pranayama* constitute the third and fourth limbs of yoga. They require physical control and mental discipline in order that the body may be mastered and its desires tamed.

Mastery of the first four limbs leads the student to the higher, 'internal' limbs, called *samyama* in Sanskrit. *Pratyahara*, the fifth limb, requires withdrawal from the distractions of the outside world by focusing on the soul. The sixth limb is *dharana*, meaning concentration. The aim here is to focus

VISUALISING YOUR CHAKRAS

According to yogic belief, seven energy centres or 'chakras' span the body from the base of the spine to the head, linking the mind with the body. Each chakra is depicted as a lotus flower, has a particular colour, which follow those of the rainbow, and is associated with a specific psychological or spiritual function such as love or survival.

MEDITATIVE FOCUS
To concentrate on the associations linked to a particular chakra, imagine it superimposed on your body, its colour glowing strongly.

Crown or *sahasrara* chakra. Related to oneness and wisdom. Colour: violet.

Brow or *ajna* chakra. Related to clarity of thought and mental agility. Colour: indigo.

Throat or *vishuddi* chakra. Related to creativity. Colour: bright blue.

Heart or *anahata* chakra. Related to feelings of love and peace. Colour: green.

Solar plexus or *manipura* chakra. Related to power and will. Colour: yellow.

Sacral or *svadisthana* chakra. Related to sexuality and pleasure. Colour: orange.

Base or *muladhara* chakra. Related to survival and grounding. Colour: red.

Warming up for

Yoga and T'ai Chi

These forms of exercise promote mental focus and physical flexibility. To prepare for a session, it is important not only to stretch and to warm up all the major muscle groups of the body, but also to calm and focus the mind with meditation.

Start your yoga preparation with a period of meditation to calm and prepare your mind. Begin by sitting in a comfortable upright position with your shoulders relaxed. Close your eyes and try to concentrate on the sound of your breathing. Breathe slowly and rhythmically, without force. Counting your breath can help to divert your mind from external troubling thoughts. Count in sets of five in-breaths, focusing on the physical sensation of the breath in the nostrils as it enters the body.

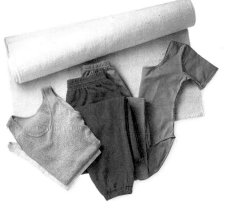

EXERCISE ESSENTIALS
Wear comfortable exercise clothing in breathable fabrics. A mat or a towel will be useful for yoga floor work.

STRETCHES TO WARM UP YOUR MUSCLES

After about 10 minutes of meditation, you can move on to a physical warm-up. It is important to enter into yoga gradually, so always begin with a series of exercises and stretches that increase the mobility of the joints and warm and stretch the muscles. The warm-up will help to release any tension stored in the body, allowing a full range of movement in the session itself. This reduces the risk of injury and will enable you to benefit fully from your yoga session.

Combine the stretches shown here with those featured in Chapter 5 (see pages 94-136) to create a warm-up that begins at the top of your head and works down towards your feet. This will give the sensation of tension dropping away.

Try to stretch to the same point when you repeat the stretch on the other side

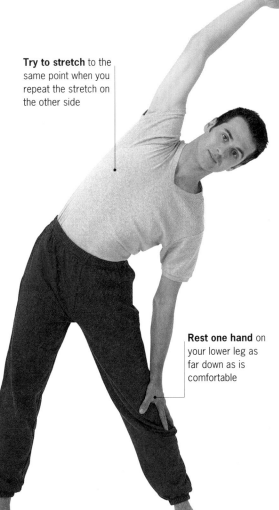

Rest one hand on your lower leg as far down as is comfortable

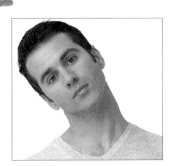

NECK STRETCH
Tilt your head slowly towards your right shoulder, then slowly return it to the centre before tilting to the left. Repeat five times.

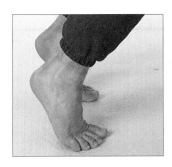

FOOT FLEXOR
Hold onto the back of a chair for support. With a bend in your knees, slowly lift your heels off the floor; then down. Repeat four times.

SIDE STRETCH
Stand with your feet wide apart. Slide your left hand down your left leg. At the same time extend your right arm over your head to the left as far as you can, following with your upper body. Do not lean forwards. Hold the stretch 10–20 seconds, then slowly return to the start position. Repeat the stretch to the other side.

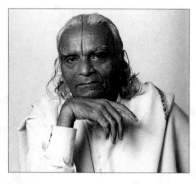

PRESENT-DAY GURU
BKS Iyengar is recognised as the world's foremost authority on the science of yoga.

Origins

Now in his old age, BKS Iyengar has devoted his life to the study of yoga. Honoured for his services to the future of yoga by the Government of India, he has systemised more than 2000 postures and breathing techniques. He has worked extensively on the therapeutic benefits of yoga, adapting many postures to make them more accessible and beneficial to people with disabilities.

Over the centuries, many different schools of yoga have developed, each placing a varying emphasis on different aspects of yogic practice. One of the most popular forms in the West, and an easily accessible form for the novice, is Hatha yoga. The Sanskrit word *Hatha* can be broken into two elements: 'ha' meaning sun, and 'tha' meaning moon. This pairing of opposites represents the yogic ideal of balance between the mind and body, and between active energy and passive relaxation. When neither of these aspects outweighs the other, we perform better in our day-to-day lives and experience optimum levels of health.

Hatha yoga takes the physical body as a starting point, emphasising posture (asanas) and breathing (pranayama) as a means of achieving health. A practical system of concentration and mental discipline is used to bring the body into various postures, which strengthen the muscles, correct misalignments of the back and limbs, massage the internal organs and encourage a state of relaxation and emotional tranquillity.

the mind in order to stop it becoming distracted or wandering. This leads to the seventh limb, called *dhayana* or meditation. The final sutra that can be achieved is the trance state, *samadhi*, which is the state of heightened consciousness that can lead to ultimate mental freedom.

BASIC YOGA MOVEMENTS

Yoga exercises involve a variety of postures and positions – standing, sitting, lying or kneeling. The following exercises offer a sample of some of the many postures, or asanas, which can improve your flexibility, muscle tone and balance.

RISHI'S POSTURE

1 *Begin in a standing position with your feet together. Transfer your weight on to your left leg. Bend your right leg at the knee without moving the position of your thigh. Take hold of your right foot with your right hand and draw it up towards your bottom.*

2 *From Rishi's Posture, inhale and lift your left arm up above your head. Hold the position, look straight ahead and maintain relaxed breathing.*

3 *Gently stretch your right foot away from your bottom and shift your weight forwards. Relax into the posture and maintain breathing. Repeat using your left leg.*

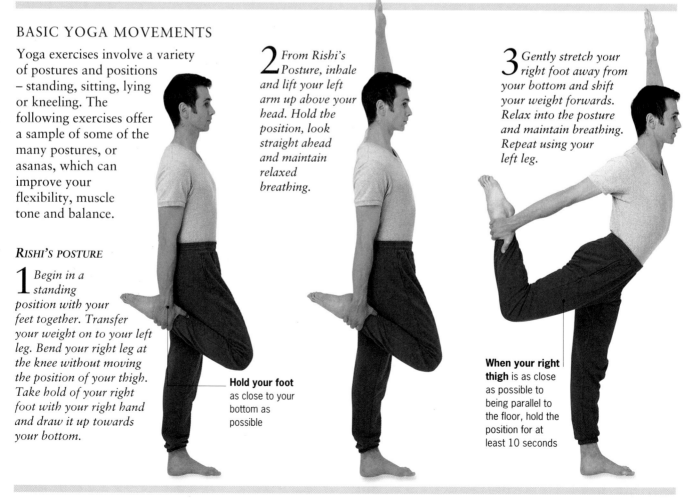

Hold your foot as close to your bottom as possible

When your right thigh is as close as possible to being parallel to the floor, hold the position for at least 10 seconds

How yoga improves flexibility and tone

A yoga routine will often begin with breathing exercises called pranayama. Focusing intently on the breath in this way screens out extraneous thoughts or anxieties and connects the mind with the body, allowing the participant's potential life energy (the prana) to be accessed.

Pranayama strengthens the respiratory muscles, calms the nervous system and relaxes the body in order to prepare it for the asanas. Good breath control is essential to maintain stable postures during a yoga routine and can be extremely effective in helping to cope with stressful situations. When inhaling, you should visualise the body drawing in life energy; with each exhalation, imagine you are expelling waste products and toxins, breathing them onto a fire which burns them away. Combining breath control with the various yoga postures revitalises both the body and mind.

Asanas are the physical expression of, as well as being the practical route to achieving, the unification of body and spirit which is the aim of all the various forms of yoga. Asanas are stretching postures, performed without force in a slow, relaxed manner. They are designed to release tension from the joints, muscles, ligaments and tendons, as well as to tone up the internal systems of the body.

Although its movements are non-violent and slow, yoga nonetheless provides a thorough muscular work-out, which improves tone, strength and flexibility. The stretches

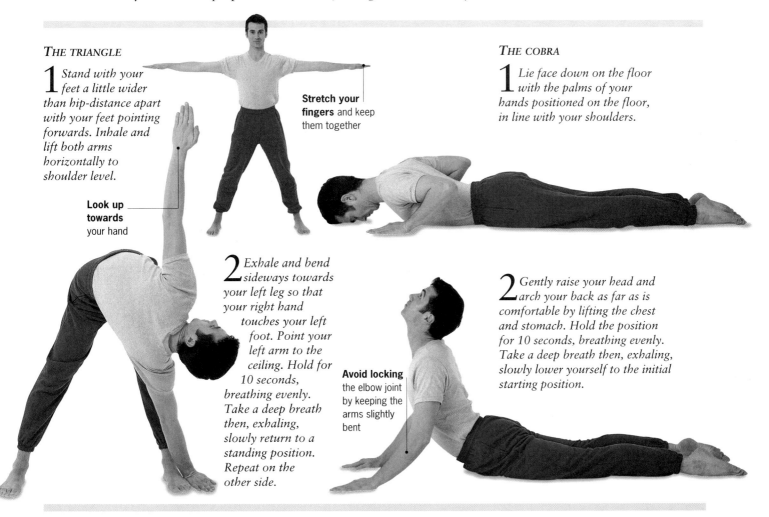

THE TRIANGLE

1 *Stand with your feet a little wider than hip-distance apart with your feet pointing forwards. Inhale and lift both arms horizontally to shoulder level.*

Stretch your fingers and keep them together

Look up towards your hand

2 *Exhale and bend sideways towards your left leg so that your right hand touches your left foot. Point your left arm to the ceiling. Hold for 10 seconds, breathing evenly. Take a deep breath then, exhaling, slowly return to a standing position. Repeat on the other side.*

THE COBRA

1 *Lie face down on the floor with the palms of your hands positioned on the floor, in line with your shoulders.*

2 *Gently raise your head and arch your back as far as is comfortable by lifting the chest and stomach. Hold the position for 10 seconds, breathing evenly. Take a deep breath then, exhaling, slowly lower yourself to the initial starting position.*

Avoid locking the elbow joint by keeping the arms slightly bent

Balanced breath

According to traditional belief, the pranayama breathing technique of inhaling through one nostril and exhaling through the other unites the opposing sides of our nature and eliminates imbalance between them. The right nostril is associated with activity and rationality, and the left with our passive emotional side. In Ayurvedic medicine, this technique is used as a means of balancing the doshas (see page 46).

are static, as opposed to the bouncing or 'ballistic' stretches which may be found in some forms of exercise, and which can put stress on the joints and skeletal structure. Ideally, an asana should be held for at least 20–30 seconds, although it may take some practice to achieve this length of time. This means that the muscle is held long enough in the stretch to relax and increase in length slightly. As a result, the regular practice of asanas over a period of time often leads to a longer, leaner musculature, rather than simply increasing muscle bulk, as is the case in some forms of aerobic exercise. While one muscle is stretching, another is having to remain contracted in order to maintain steady posture. This static contraction also helps to develop physical strength and endurance.

Manoeuvring into and out of each position smoothly can be difficult at first. As the exercises become more familiar, communication from mind to body also improves, resulting in improved balance and co-ordination.

If a joint is slightly out of place and is not realigned properly, the muscles and tendons around it become tense and knotted as the body attempts to stabilise the problem area. This results in stiffness and pain. Practising asanas can correct misalignments, freeing up movement. The concentrated training both muscles and joints receive also contributes to increased flexibility.

Yoga can be practised either in a class or by yourself at home. If you are a beginner, it is advisable to attend a class run by a properly trained yoga teacher. If you are practising at home, make some time for yourself at a suitable period during the day when there are no distractions – first thing in the morning is ideal. It is important not to practise yoga on a full stomach, so allow plenty of time between meals. Wear something comfortable and loose-fitting so you can move freely, and ensure the room is clean and has a good supply of fresh air. You do not need special equipment for the practice of yoga although a mat can be helpful for some postures.

ENDING A SESSION

To finish a yoga session, choose positions which gently stretch the muscles and can then be held to allow body and mind to completely relax. The child pose increases flexibility in the hips and has a calming effect, while the corpse pose is so relaxing it can induce sleep.

THE CHILD POSE

1 *Kneel, sitting on your heels. Keeping your back straight, stretch your body upwards. Link your fingers with palms facing front and gently raise your arms above your head. Release your fingers, keeping palms facing front.*

Relax your arms by your sides with palms facing upwards

2 *Bring your arms down to your thighs. Take a deep breath and, exhaling, slowly fold your body down over your legs until your forehead is gently touching the floor. Hold the position for about a minute, then take another deep breath and, exhaling, slowly return to the start position.*

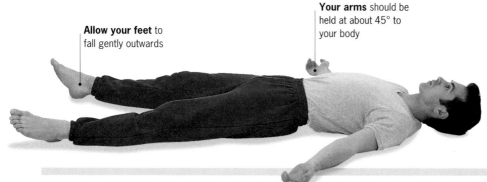

Allow your feet to fall gently outwards

Your arms should be held at about 45° to your body

THE CORPSE POSE

This position can be held for 5 minutes at the start and end of a session, and can also be practised as a relaxation technique between the more difficult postures of a yoga session. Lie flat on your back with your arms and legs apart. Close your eyes and lie still. Relax your body and feel the contact of your back with the floor. Breathe evenly.

Toning Up With T'ai Chi

The slow, controlled movements of t'ai chi have been practised for centuries by the Chinese as a means of exercising the body and focusing the mind to promote health and longevity.

T'ai chi is formally classed as a martial art, but is practised today mainly for its beneficial effect on emotional and physical well-being. Sometimes described as an 'internal martial art', it differs from other Eastern martial arts forms, such as judo and aikido, because it is non-combative and uses internal techniques such as breath control, visualisation and channelling of energy, to achieve psychological as well as physical strength. Although other martial arts are also good for toning up and developing muscular strength, stamina and speed of reaction, t'ai chi's focus on more spiritual aspects makes it ideal for anyone.

THE HISTORY OF T'AI CHI
According to tradition, the 13th-century Taoist priest, Zhang San Feng, created t'ai chi after witnessing a fight between a crane

BASIC T'AI CHI MOVEMENTS

The movements of t'ai chi are slow, continuous and purposeful, often working through a designated series of flowing forms or postures, which together create what is called a 'set'. Start each posture by standing with the feet slightly wider than hip distance. Bend the knees a little and focus on your back to maintain an upright, central position that feels natural to the spine. The aim is to perform each stance with strength and power in the legs, whilst the shoulders remain relaxed and free from tension.

SINGLE WHIP

1 *Put your weight on your left leg, and keep your right leg slightly bent and soft. Make the shape of a bird's beak with your right hand and place the fingers of the left hand lightly on the right wrist.*

2 *Take a wide step back with your right leg and shift your weight forwards, bending your left knee. Stretch your left arm outwards with the fingers pointing up and the right arm backwards with the fingers pointing down.*

Keep your back straight but not tensed

Keep the bent knee soft and not locked

and a snake. He was surprised to see that the bird's calm and graceful defensive movements proved a strong match for the explosive strikes of the snake and was thus inspired to develop a martial art which took as its philosophy the idea of using minimum force to combat maximum strength. Since its foundation, t'ai chi has evolved into many different styles, some emphasising combat and others completely given over to improving health.

The full name of the art, 't'ai chi chuan', comes from the Chinese *'t'ai chi'* meaning 'cosmos', and *'chuan fa'* meaning 'way of the fist', in revealing its roots as a fighting style. However, one of the most popular forms practised today is the Yang style developed by Yang Deng Fu (1883–1936), who eliminated many of the more aggressive actions – such as jumps, kicks and straight punches – in order to emphasise the health aspect of t'ai chi chuan. With this move away from the martial aspect, many practitioners drop the reference to combat and simply call this style 't'ai chi'.

DID YOU KNOW?

The relaxing effect of t'ai chi on the mind and its beneficial effects on physical health have prompted insurance companies in Germany to pay their clients greater dividends if they learn t'ai chi or chi kung – a related martial art.

How t'ai chi works

The graceful and controlled movements of t'ai chi help to stimulate the flow of energy ('chi') around the body, along the channels also used in acupuncture. Regular practice replenishes lost energy, improving both your mental and physical shape.

In traditional Chinese medicine, the energy system is considered the basic foundation of health, upon which all other bodily systems are built. If our energy is blocked, we therefore become ill. T'ai chi clears energy blockages, thus helping to prevent serious illnesses, such as hypertension, asthma and rheumatism. T'ai chi is widely recognised as

PARTING THE HORSE'S MANE

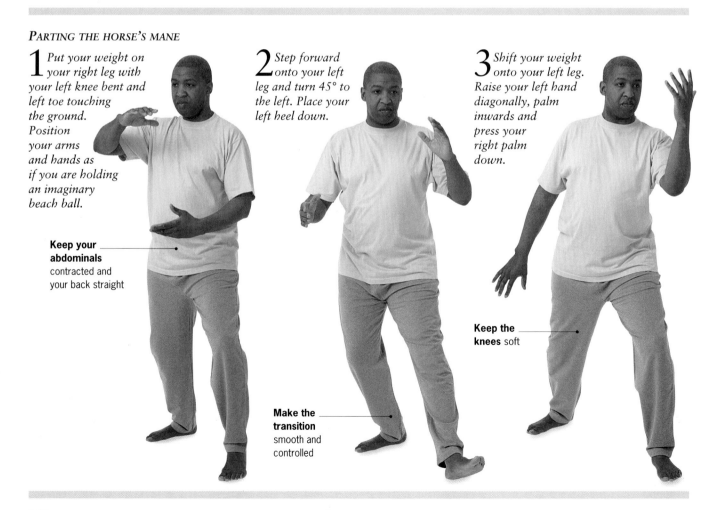

1 *Put your weight on your right leg with your left knee bent and left toe touching the ground. Position your arms and hands as if you are holding an imaginary beach ball.*

Keep your abdominals contracted and your back straight

2 *Step forward onto your left leg and turn 45° to the left. Place your left heel down.*

Make the transition smooth and controlled

3 *Shift your weight onto your left leg. Raise your left hand diagonally, palm inwards and press your right palm down.*

Keep the knees soft

a stress-reduction therapy and for increasing mobility in the elderly. It may even be helpful in the prevention of cancer.

The concept of yin and yang is an important part of t'ai chi. The two words signify opposing pairs of forces – for example masculine and feminine, light and dark – which govern the universe. Imbalance between these forces results in physical or emotional illness. T'ai chi restores balance through movements which alternate between hard (the yang or masculine principle) and soft (the yin or feminine principle) to promote calm, mental clarity and equilibrium.

How t'ai chi improves toning

Each position in t'ai chi is achieved through smooth linking movements which may look effortless but require great control. This develops muscular strength in the legs as they balance, bend, straighten and change direction or height. The slow pace of movement accentuates the effect of the exercise and a lot of leg power is needed to hold the deep stance required. Other physical bene-

fits include increased mobility of the spine and flexibility in the joints. If practised correctly t'ai chi can also prevent or relieve knee injury, which US studies have shown to be the most common and disabling form of joint problems.

T'ai chi benefits the body as a whole, not only toning the muscles which are visible to the eye but also benefiting internal muscles and organs. Breath control exercises slow respiration and maximise the energy derived from breathing. T'ai chi also improves the function of the digestive system, maximising the energy we obtain from the minimum amount of food. Food is converted into energy rather than mass, benefiting those who wish to lose excess weight.

As with any form of exercise, it is important to include a warm-up or preparation period before a t'ai chi session. This should include gentle movements that loosen the joints and warm and stretch the muscles; but of equal importance are breathing and concentration exercises to focus the mind and aid relaxation.

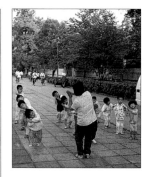

STARTING YOUNG
Regular exercise is an integral part of Chinese life from an early age. Because the movements of t'ai chi are slow and deliberate, it is suitable for all ages, from children, when it encourages balance and coordination, to old people, when it can maintain joint mobility and clarity of mind.

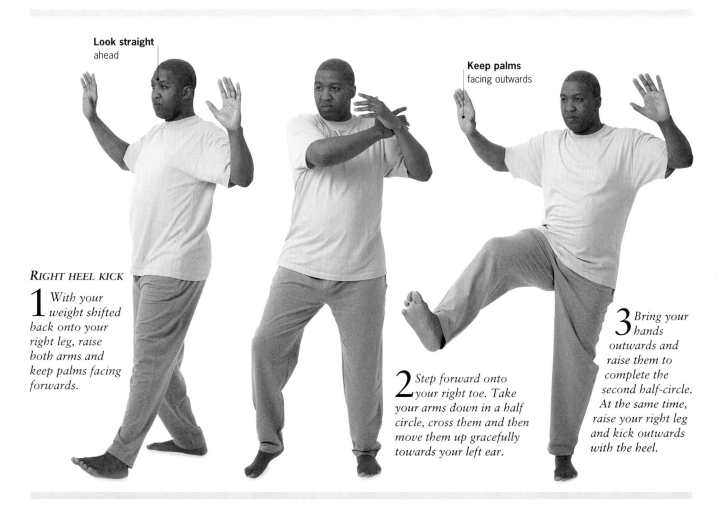

Look straight ahead

Keep palms facing outwards

RIGHT HEEL KICK

1 *With your weight shifted back onto your right leg, raise both arms and keep palms facing forwards.*

2 *Step forward onto your right toe. Take your arms down in a half circle, cross them and then move them up gracefully towards your left ear.*

3 *Bring your hands outwards and raise them to complete the second half-circle. At the same time, raise your right leg and kick outwards with the heel.*

Dancing to Get in Shape

To dance is a natural instinct; it provides an opportunity to explore the body's creative potential, to exercise the muscles, joints and respiratory system, and to focus the mind.

Dance is our primary form of physical expression, allowing body, mind and spirit to work together creatively. It can be a highly disciplined, technical art or it can be enjoyed simply as a healthy activity and a great way to get in shape. With such a variety of different types of dance, it is possible for anyone, whatever age, to find one which suits them and their personal needs. Different forms of dance offer a variety of shaping-up benefits; one style may be particularly beneficial for toning the legs or the waist, while another may strengthen the lower back or stomach.

BALLET

Ballet originated in the royal courts of France and Italy during the 16th century, developing from the spectacular performances which had entertained the ruling

BASIC BALLET MOVEMENTS

Ballet offers wonderful physical benefits, no matter what your fitness level. The following exercises are based on classical ballet movements and can help you to strengthen your muscles and acquire a more graceful posture.

PLIÉ SIDE STRETCH

This exercise gently warms up the body and is particularly good for toning the inner thighs and improving balance. Regular practice improves posture by preventing slouching and relieving tension in the lower back.

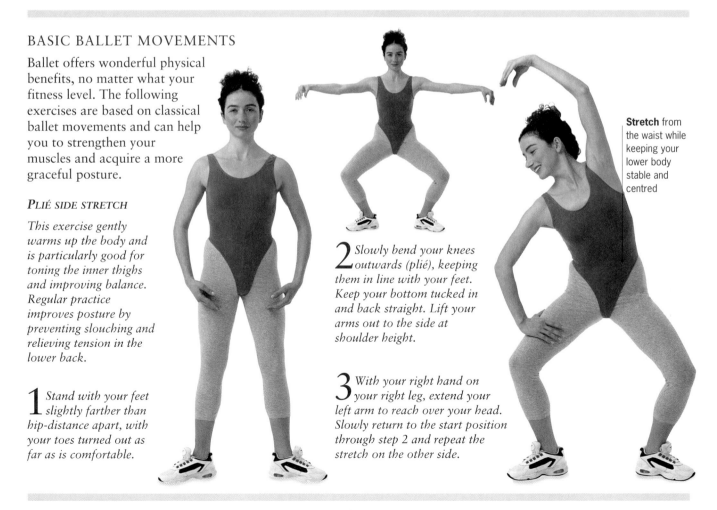

1 *Stand with your feet slightly farther than hip-distance apart, with your toes turned out as far as is comfortable.*

2 *Slowly bend your knees outwards (plié), keeping them in line with your feet. Keep your bottom tucked in and back straight. Lift your arms out to the side at shoulder height.*

3 *With your right hand on your right leg, extend your left arm to reach over your head. Slowly return to the start position through step 2 and repeat the stretch on the other side.*

Stretch from the waist while keeping your lower body stable and centred

classes since the Middle Ages. The steps were derived from the social dances of the time and emphasised restraint and decorum in contrast to the athleticism of modern ballet technique. During the 17th century, the emphasis began to shift and dance was regarded as an increasingly serious form of art, with set steps and gestures which had to be performed correctly.

How ballet improves flexibility and tone

Ballet can be used to tone distinct areas of the body. Try to perform the movements in a smooth, controlled manner, without jerking, and make sure you warm up before you start. Remember to wear comfortable clothing that doesn't restrict movement. It is probably worth investing in ballet slippers although you may dance barefoot.

Ballet can either be taken to the extreme perfection of the professional dancer, or enjoyed simply as a way to improve health and fitness. The many different moods and styles of ballet cater for all tastes and levels

Origins

Classical ballet owes much to composer Jean-Baptiste Lully (1632–87). Lully first emerged as a young dancer and violinist in the court of the 'Sun King' Louis XIV. Louis was a passionate court dancer and in 1661 founded a Royal Academy of Dancing which established many of ballet's enduring traditions. Throughout his career Lully composed ballet music which did much to popularise the dance form.

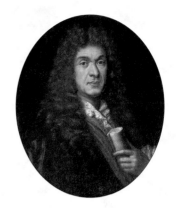

THE KING'S COMPOSER
A favourite of Louis XIV, Lully wrote music specifically designed to accompany ballet steps.

of fitness. Ballet is a highly effective way of improving overall flexibility and muscle tone, it can help to develop coordination and balance, and will do much to improve your posture in your everyday life.

continued on page 150

HIP ROTATIONS

This exercise improves posture by stabilising the pelvis and increasing flexibility in the hips, and also helps to strengthen and tone the outer thighs.

Keep your body
in a straight line to protect the lower back

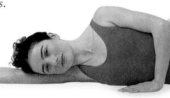

1 *Lie on your right side with your legs together. Rest your head on your right* arm and place your left arm in front of your torso to stabilise your body.

Pull in the abdominals
to stabilise your pelvis

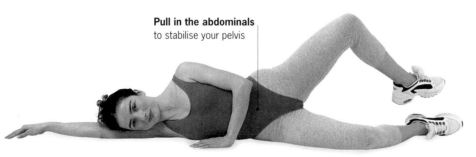

2 *Raise your left leg in a parallel position. Next, rotate the leg from the hip so that your knee is pointing to the ceiling and your toe is pointing down.*

Repeat 10 times and then turn onto your opposite side and repeat the exercise with the other leg.

Return to start position
very slowly

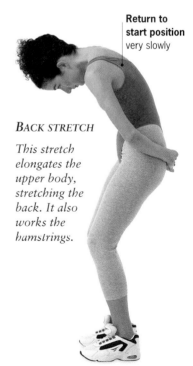

BACK STRETCH

This stretch elongates the upper body, stretching the back. It also works the hamstrings.

Stand tall to start, with your feet hip-width apart. Clasp your hands behind your back and, with a slight bend at the knees, round your back forwards. Gently straighten.

The Ballet Teacher

Ballet is more accessible than many people think and is a good way to get fit and have fun at the same time. Dance classes are available for all ages and cater for all levels of ability, from those with a background in dance to complete beginners.

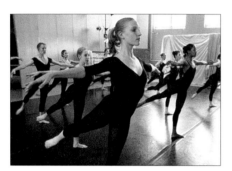

CLASS ACT
Learning ballet in a class provides a framework for self-expression, physical discipline, an elegant posture and graceful movements.

BALLET FOR EVERYONE
Your peak flexibility is at around 10 years of age, but it is never too late to start ballet lessons. Dance can help to improve your self-image and confidence.

The ballet teacher provides technical supervision and stylistic guidance as well as safeguarding the student from physical injury. A positive rapport with a teacher can also help students to learn to interpret their emotions through movement.

What qualifications must a ballet teacher have?

Teachers must hold a recognised qualification in order to teach the various disciplines of modern or classical ballet; many will also have experience as a dancer which they can draw upon. In the UK the two most established ballet organisations are the Royal Academy of Dance (RAD) and the Imperial Society of Teachers of Dancing (ISTD). Most ballet teachers will be approved by one of these two organisations and teach according to their exam syllabuses. Other recognised and respected ways of teaching ballet include the Cecchetti and the Russian methods.

Who can do it?

Ballet is open to all ages and abilities: it is not necessary to have danced since you were a child, have a sylph-like figure or be super-fit. The pleasure of dancing and creating positive energy through a sequence of steps can be achieved at any level of ability. If you are unused to balletic movements, do not worry if you find the steps difficult at first – do only what you are capable of without forcing your body and you will find that your flexibility and strength gradually increase.

Are there any contraindications?

If you are pregnant, have high blood pressure, a balance disorder or joint complaint, such as arthritis, you should check with your doctor whether ballet is an appropriate form of exercise. It can actually be beneficial for certain conditions, for example, children suffering from sclerosis can sometimes avoid permanent curvature of the spine through taking ballet lessons.

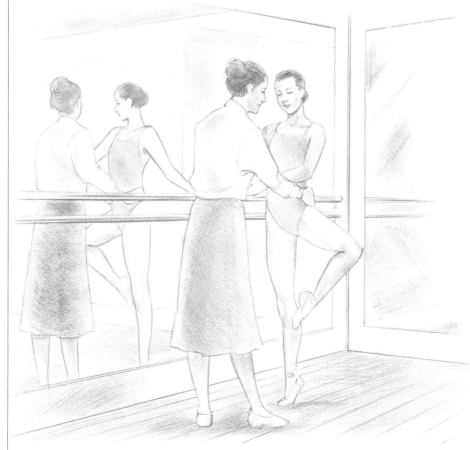

What to expect from a dance class

Classes are widely available for all levels of proficiency, often classified as beginner, intermediate or advanced. If you are new to dance, then the beginner's class will be most appropriate, being the least complicated and strenuous. However, many classes are of a 'general' standard where the teacher will adapt to the needs of the class and offer relevant alternatives for individuals of different abilities within the group. Most classes for adults are 'freestyle' and do not follow a dance exam syllabus.

Ballet classes, like most forms of work-out, will always include a warm-up section: this readies you for activity by getting the blood circulating to all the systems of the body, especially the major muscle groups and joints. In ballet, the warm-up always includes a sequence of exercises performed at the 'barre' which help to mobilise the joints, build strength in the muscles and provide the groundwork for the more dynamic floor exercises.

This is the main part of the ballet class and is divided into sections; graceful and slow arm movements ('port de bras'); technique work for the legs and arms; more dynamic jumps ('allegro'), turns ('pirouette') and large jump sequences ('grande allegro'). These sections are then used to create a short routine. The cooling down period at the end of the class is as important as the warm-up. Stretching exercises are repeated and you may be asked to hold positions for a few moments more than at the beginning of the class, or extend the leg a little further; this is because the muscles will have greater flexibility and strength after they have been thoroughly exercised. After the stretches your heart rate and breathing should slow again.

The teacher will lead by demonstrating each movement carefully before the class performs it. He or she will also offer individual guidance to students throughout the class to ensure that posture is correct and the right groups of muscles are being worked.

What are the benefits of ballet?

Dance can be appreciated at many levels, from finely tuned professionalism to the enjoyment of dancing around the house to your favourite piece of music. Ballet offers excellent cardiovascular training and if the exercises are performed regularly, it can significantly improve the health of the heart and lungs. The disciplined technique of ballet improves motor skills such as coordination and balance, as well as developing the muscular strength, flexibility and endurance which result in a well-defined physique, good posture and a graceful way of moving.

Exercising the body in a creative way can also achieve very positive results for your personal well-being: it is a great way to relax and express suppressed emotions. Dance can be a release from everyday activities and an opportunity for you to become more aware of your body and explore the way it can move. Set steps form the basis of any form of dance but can also be individually interpreted providing a therapeutic outlet for emotional expression which can ultimately improve self-confidence and lead to a more outgoing personality.

WHAT YOU CAN DO AT HOME

It is important to translate the benefits of ballet from the class into every aspect of your life. The heightened bodily awareness that ballet brings can be used to make adjustments to your posture in everyday situations. Make a point of stopping at various intervals in your day and try the following exercises. Remember that strong abdominal muscles and a strong back help to support the whole of the body and keep the centre of balance stable. This will relieve pressure on the lower back and is especially important if you are sedentary for much of the day.

POSTURE PROMOTION
Pull yourself up to your full height. Imagine a piece of string is connected from the centre point on the top of your head, right down through the centre of your body. Imagine this string to be 'pulling' and 'lifting' you upwards. Make sure your shoulders are not raised or tense and think about your back and abdomen.

BACK STRETCH
From the standing position, bend your knees and fold forwards from your waist. Keep your back and neck as straight as possible and feel your lower back releasing.

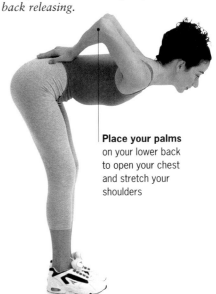

Place your palms on your lower back to open your chest and stretch your shoulders

Practising ballet requires the muscles to hold (or fixate) the body to maintain the required position, which strengthens the muscles. Simply by standing with correct balletic posture, the muscles statically contract. For example, the basic static posture (first position) tones the leg muscles by turning them out from the hips down.

When dancing a sequence of steps, a great deal of muscle work in both the lower and upper body is used. To bend, straighten, lift, turn, extend and contract requires a great deal of physical work. However, it is important in ballet that the body remain light and the movements appear effortless and airy.

Ballet is made up of a great range of movements, some focusing on graceful and lyrical sequences, which require tremendous muscle control to maintain balance, while others are quick and explosive. This trains the muscles to work at various speeds, improving reaction time and coordination. Ballet exercises strengthen muscles without building excess bulk and are wonderful for producing long, lean lines.

The stretching exercises which form an important part of a ballet work-out, develop flexibility of the muscles and increase the range of movement possible in the joints, allowing the body to extend to its full capability. If dancing for health, aim to develop flexibility through slow, static type stretches. Do not 'bounce' stretches and make sure you warm up properly.

Although people generally 'know' what correct posture is, they are unaware of how they hold their bodies day-to-day, unless consciously thinking about it. This can result in habitual stoops or slouching. The classically upright stance – with shoulders back and stomach in – is held by trained dancers at all times because their bodies 'remember' to do so. Ballet exercises sensitise this physical memory, making the body more responsive and helping us to become aware of our posture in everyday life.

BASIC SALSA MOVEMENTS

Salsa is ideal for a couple who want to exercise together and like to dance. Here, we show you a few basic steps but you will probably need to join a class to get a real 'feel' for the dance. It offers a good cardiovascular work-out for both partners, with the woman's hips and stomach working extra hard when turning.

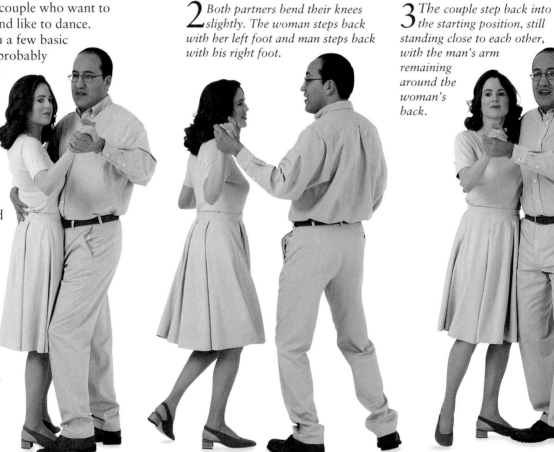

1 *This is the start position for all steps. With backs held straight, both partners stand close together. The man places his right arm around the woman's waist. The woman's right hand rests lightly in the man's left hand.*

2 *Both partners bend their knees slightly. The woman steps back with her left foot and man steps back with his right foot.*

3 *The couple step back into the starting position, still standing close to each other, with the man's arm remaining around the woman's back.*

SALSA

Based on the old Cuban rhythm known as *Son*, the Salsa rhythm was invented by Caribbean (mainly Cuban) musicians in New York in the 1960s and 70s. It is danced in a couple and the man leads the woman in a tight, smooth, sensuous progression of turns, which can include more spectacular, arm-spinning and multi-turn figures. The soles of the feet remain close to the ground, the knees often slightly bent. The grace of the dance is in the movement of the hips.

Salsa for fitness

The muscles used in this dance are those of the thighs and hips, so it is an exceptionally good exercise for the legs. The waistline also benefits from the constant twisting of the hips. The overall speed of movement and the fast tempo of the music make salsa an excellent form of aerobic exercise.

In recent years the popularity of salsa has rocketed as people have discovered what a wonderfully social exercise activity it is. Classes are readily available in most large cities, and although the more advanced steps can be quite complex and intricate, most people find the basic steps quick and easy to acquire. Once you have mastered a few simple movements there are many nightclubs and dance events where you will be able to practise your new skills.

FLAMENCO

Flamenco had its beginnings in Andalusia, a region of southern Spain. This area has long been a cultural melting pot, with music and dance influenced by the many groups of people who settled there. It was in this atmosphere of cultural diversity, towards the end of the 18th century, that a local gypsy (*gitano*) form of folk music and dance called flamenco rose to prominence in the area, and now enjoys popularity not only all over Spain but also in many other parts of the world.

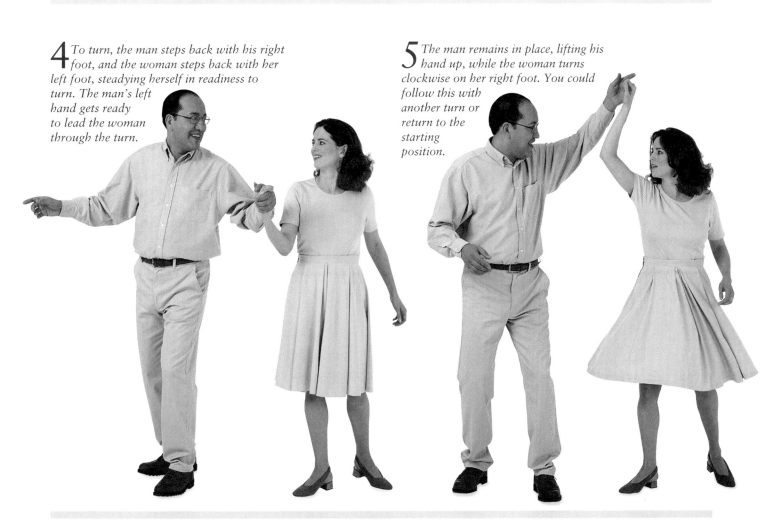

4 To turn, the man steps back with his right foot, and the woman steps back with her left foot, steadying herself in readiness to turn. The man's left hand gets ready to lead the woman through the turn.

5 The man remains in place, lifting his hand up, while the woman turns clockwise on her right foot. You could follow this with another turn or return to the starting position.

In flamenco, the language of the body is concerned with the expression of the intense emotions and fundamental forces which govern our lives, such as love, hate, death, fate and morality. The communication of these feelings evokes powerful reactions in both the performers – musicians, singers and dancers – and the audience. Flamenco classes offer an intimate space in which people are able to express freely these emotions through the passionate movements of the dance. This is in keeping with the traditional context of flamenco, which is quite intimate and not essentially about performing to a large audience.

In Spain flamenco performances are often spontaneous, taking place in the family home or in taverns, with members of the gathering simply taking turns to sing, play or dance. The audience are thus intended to participate and share in the experience, not critically observe. This intimacy differentiates flamenco from many other forms of dance. It is not an extrovert performance, using expansive spaces or spectacularly acrobatic moves.

There are no specific age boundaries for taking up flamenco. More important than a youthful physique is maturity and experience of the joys and pains that life brings, which can usually only be acquired with age. This has meant that some of the greatest flamenco dancers have reached the height of their careers in their 60s! Although you may choose not to perform some of the more vigorous steps, the arm movements

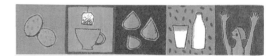

SUPER SHAPER

One of the most effective forms of shaping-up dances is the Twist which first emerged in the 1960s. Some people have suggested the dance originated as a stylised version of the way rock 'n' roll singers swung their hips. It was very easy to learn: people were taught to move their feet as if they were trying to stub out a cigarette, and move their hips as if they were drying the sweat off their back with a towel – and there was no need for a partner. The Twist was, and still is, a great way to lose weight; in the first year of the Twist craze Chubby Checker, who recorded the song 'The Twist' in 1960, lost 16 kilos (35 lbs) performing the dance to his hit record.

and basic footwork can continue to be performed as you get older, and will help to maintain good strength and flexibility.

Flamenco for fitness

Flamenco dance is not only expressive, it can also be a great way to get fit and stay in shape. There is a strong emphasis on maintaining an upright position. Women should hold the back in a slightly arched posture, while men should give the impression of height through a straight spine. This requires both the muscles of the back and the opposing muscle group, the abdominals, to work hard.

A great deal of strength and endurance is required in the leg muscles for the characteristic stamping action (*zapato*). This step demands so much physical force that it was originally a step performed solely by men, and the women's dance still places a greater emphasis on hand and arm movements. Because the legs include some of the body's largest muscles, they demand more oxygen to function. This kind of aerobic training helps to burn excess fat, although a slim or youthful figure is not considered necessary in order to dance the flamenco well.

Many of the women's steps incorporate arm, wrist and hand movements, revealing the influence of traditional Arabic dance, as

FLAMENCO AND THE GYPSIES
Andalusian gypsies celebrate festivals with singing and flamenco dancing. The true gypsy flamenco is never choreographed but emerges spontaneously from the heart.

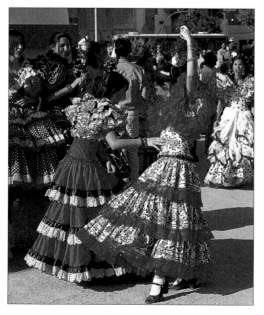

NATIONAL DANCES

Many nationalities all over the world celebrate their culture with a form of dance that has been handed down from generation to generation and is often performed at a particular time of year. Many are linked to traditional folk tales and some include ancient rituals. For example, in England part of the Morris dancing tradition involves teams of dancers visiting each village in the local area in turn in order to bring good luck. Other aspects of Morris dancing celebrate fertility. For example, the Maypole dance was traditionally an intricate form of courting for young village men and women.

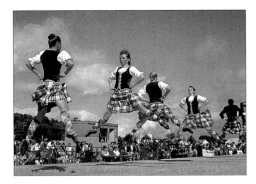

HIGHLAND DANCING
Traditional Scottish dancing from the Highland regions requires a high level of fitness, good flexibility and very strong inner thigh muscles.

the Koran forbids a woman to show her legs. For example, finger snapping (*pitos*) and rhythmic hand clapping (*palmas*) are important accompaniments to the dance. This helps to develop greater flexibility in the wrist and shoulder joints.

BELLY DANCING

Belly dancing originated in the Middle East but variations can be found all over the world, from Southern Europe to North Africa. Contemporary belly dancing popular in the West is considered by many to have originated in Egypt. However, many of the movements of this dance have also been influenced by Indian, Turkish and other Middle Eastern forms of dancing.

Traditionally, in Middle Eastern countries, people were exposed to music and dancing in every aspect of their lives, regardless of age, fitness or social class. Dancers of both sexes performed in private at celebrations such as weddings or the birth of a child, as part of religious worship, and in public – even in the streets. Consequently, dance was enjoyed instinctively and participated in without inhibitions. Although the style of belly dancing has changed over the years, its celebratory qualities still remain today and many people, from different cultural backgrounds, find personal fulfilment in such unrestricted, exuberant and sensual movement.

Although originally a dance performed by women for other women, nowadays belly dancing can be practised and enjoyed by

both sexes. It is traditional for men in the Middle East to dance using many belly dancing movements, and men still perform the dance at social functions, including religious festivals. In contrast to the undulating style of the female dance, the men's movements are more athletic.

The notion of maintaining a free spirit and enhancing self-expression is integral to belly dancing and is the primary impulse and energy source of the dance. The distinctive rhythmic patterns of Middle Eastern music provide the atmospheric backdrop to which moves are improvised, freely interpreting the mood of the music.

Belly dancing for fitness

Belly dancing emphasises a downward movement of the body, as opposed to the upward lift which characterises ballet. The feet remain grounded in most steps, bearing the weight down towards the floor, while the hips and middle section of the body are the main focus of the dance and are most vigorously exercised. The dance is expanded and given dynamism by the expressive movements of the arms and hands.

As the middle section of the body strives for maximum movement, the muscles in this region receive a thorough work-out. Moving the hips in the characteristic circular action requires hard work from the muscles. As the hips perform this motion, a
continued on page 156

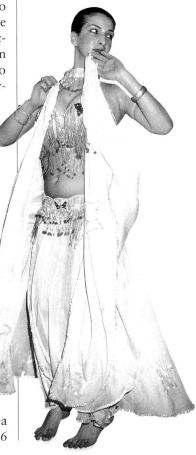

SENSUAL DANCE
Belly dancing is an uninhibited and sensual form of dance that celebrates the body. The dance form's sensuality is reflected in the evocative costumes and jewellery traditionally worn.

153

The Uninspired Exerciser

Many people begin exercise regimes with the best intentions but find it difficult to maintain interest. Shaping up and staying in shape is a long-term commitment, so it is important to choose an exercise activity about which you are genuinely enthusiastic. Remember that if you are exercising with weight loss in mind, you will need to make changes in your eating habits too.

Rosemary is a 42-year-old senior librarian with three grown-up children – Jenny, her youngest, has just left home to study at university. Up until recently Rosemary led quite an active life. She and Jenny had a very special relationship and shared much of their free time. Both keen cooks, they used to plan meals together, often experimenting with Thai and Chinese dishes. They also shared a love of evening walks and regularly walked for over an hour once or twice a week. Now that Jenny has moved out, Rosemary has a lot more free time, but isn't quite sure what to do with herself. Rosemary's husband, Gerald, has just been promoted and so often needs to work late, so Rosemary has found herself eating alone much more frequently and tends to buy convenience foods as a result.

Aware that she has slowed down over the past few months and consequently gained some excess weight, Rosemary joined an aerobics class at her local gym. However, she found it difficult to keep up with the fast pace and high-impact moves. She also can't help comparing her body to other, much younger people in the class and is feeling less positive about her self-image. She finds it hard to stay motivated about the class and often decides at the last minute not to attend, choosing to sit and watch television instead.

She has been feeling quite tired lately and has not been sleeping well. Gerald suggested a visit to the doctor but she insists that although she feels run down, she is not ill enough to bother the doctor. She misses Jenny's vitality and knows that she needs more stimulation in her own life, but increasingly she feels she has no energy to initiate any change at all.

FITNESS
Many people start to slow down as they get older and this can lead to weight gain. Keeping active will help to control weight and guard against diseases such as osteoporosis.

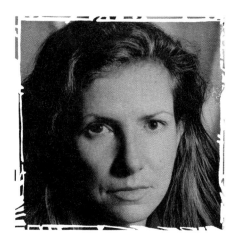

LIFESTYLE
Lack of varied stimulation in an individual's routine from outside interests and physical pursuits, can lead to lethargy, tiredness, frustration and poor fitness and motivation levels.

EMOTIONAL HEALTH
Mid-life is often a time of change, both in appearance and relationships. This may result in feelings of disorientation, dissatisfaction and poor self-esteem.

EATING HABITS
Convenience foods generally contain quite high levels of calories, and are also low in essential vitamins. It is far healthier to eat a balanced diet high in carbohydrates, fresh fruit and vegetables.

HEALTH
A degree of weight gain in middle age is normal but should be kept under control, as excess gain is physically unhealthy and contributes to an increased risk of heart disease and other serious illnesses.

WHAT SHOULD ROSEMARY DO?

Like many people, Rosemary has not given enough thought to the type of exercise she performs. To revive her interest and enthusiasm, she needs to find an activity that she genuinely enjoys. There are many forms of exercise which will achieve the same shaping-up results as Rosemary's aerobics class. She has always been fascinated with Middle Eastern culture and recently visited Turkey on holiday. Although she has never attended a dance class before, she would like to have a go at the dancing she saw while she was away.

Belly dancing classes would be ideal for Rosemary: the pace is less frenetic than aerobics, the activity is something new, and it is related to a culture in which she is interested. Belly dancing will also target the 'tummy' region which is one of Rosemary's main problem areas. Not only will she benefit physically from this type of dance but it will also be an opportunity to step out of her role as mother and wife, allowing her to release mental and physical tension through free and uninhibited movement.

Rosemary also needs to implement changes in her diet. She should try to reduce her intake of convenience foods and increase the amount of complex carbohydrates that she eats. This will make sure her body is properly fuelled for dancing.

Action Plan

FITNESS
Many forms of dance offer aerobic work-out and muscular toning equal to that gained by more conventional forms of fitness training. Choose an exercise that you enjoy so that you will not be tempted to miss sessions.

EMOTIONAL HEALTH
Find a physical outlet for your emotions which is entirely unrelated to your everyday role at work or in the home. Exercise releases 'feel good' endorphins and, especially if performed within a social environment, can help combat feelings of loneliness.

EATING HABITS
A healthy diet should go hand-in-hand with increased exercise if a shaping-up programme is to succeed. Set time aside for cooking satisfying but low-fat meals. Increase your intake of complex carbohydrates to correctly fuel your body for exercise.

HEALTH
Regular exercise reduces the risk of many serious illnesses and can boost energy levels and promote sound sleep. Choose an activity which concentrates on an area which you would particularly like to tone and strengthen. Eat more fruit and vegetables to boost the immune system.

LIFESTYLE
Exercise can be a great way to relax and de-stress as well as tone up physically. By choosing a social exercise such as dancing, you will meet like-minded people and may make new friends.

HOW THINGS TURNED OUT FOR ROSEMARY

Rosemary joined a belly dancing class, which she found through her local adult education service. Although the class is energetic, she also finds it therapeutic because it offers a safe space in which she can express herself without embarrassment. She wants to be able to do the dancing well which requires good muscle tone. For this reason, she has started going to the gym twice a week – after 40 minutes of aerobic work on the running, rowing and cycling machines, she moves to the weights room to target some of the main muscles used in belly dancing. Because she enjoys the dancing, she doesn't find motivation a problem anymore. Her body is starting to firm up and she feels much more confident about it.

Her general feeling of well-being has also increased. She has a lot more energy than previously and finds she now falls asleep easily at night. Although the exercise classes mean Rosemary is busier than she used to be, she has found time to rediscover Asian cooking. Stir-fries are quick and easy to prepare, and provide her with plenty of fresh vegetables and carbohydrates.

She has persuaded Gerald to get home early at least twice a week, and he, too, is enjoying the benefits of Rosemary's healthy eating regime, as well as her positive new outlook.

section of the mid-body has to contract. Consequently the upper and lower abdominals, the oblique muscles (at the sides of the stomach) and the muscles in the back, all receive a thorough work-out. The moves are often repeated, toning the muscles gradually through endurance. Repeated exercise of the abdominals, obliques and back muscles helps to improve the overall tone and shape of this area and also provides an excellent aerobic work-out to burn fat from all parts of the body.

The free and unrestricted movement of this oriental dance allows people to let go completely of their external concerns and anxieties, benefiting many aspects of physical health and emotional well-being, and belly dancing is generally felt to help to raise both self-esteem and confidence.

JAZZ DANCE

Jazz dance provides many of the same physical shaping-up benefits as ballet, but with a more contemporary feel and a freer style, which some people find easier to relate to. It originated in the United States, and gained widespread popularity in the 1920s during the 'Jazz Age'. Jazz dance, like the music from which it takes its name, was a Black American form developed from a mixture of elements, both African and European: aspects of ballet as well as traditional African and Latin American dances have all contributed to its style.

ROCK 'N' ROLL
The showing of the American film Rock Around The Clock *in British cinemas in the late 1950s was met by a teenaged frenzy of enthusiasm for the new dance featured – rock 'n' roll. What started as dancing in the aisles turned into riots in many cinemas, making the dance sensation unpopular with adults. The success of rock 'n' roll encouraged music promoters to try to launch other dances, the one shown here is called 'The Slug'.*

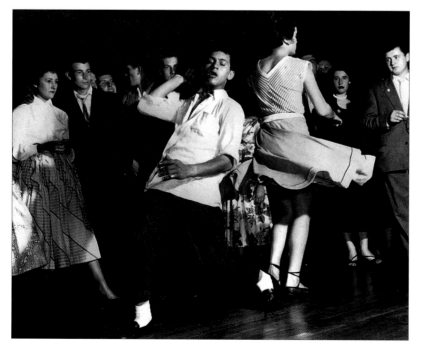

Pathway to health

Dance is no longer restricted to specialised studios: more and more adult education centres are offering exercise in evening classes and it is worth checking with your local centres to find out if any forms of dance are taught. This can be an inexpensive and sociable way of learning the foundation of the dance you are interested in and many centres may let you go along to view a session before committing to the class. The instructor will be able to advise you if the type of dance you have chosen is suitable for your needs taking into account any existing problems such as back complaints or arthritis.

Jazz dance is very flexible, offering a chance to be funky, smooth and lyrical, fast and lively, or sophisticated and stylised. The music used varies in tempo but will often include popular contemporary tracks with lyrics, as opposed to the instrumental piano music which more often accompanies ballet. The movements in jazz are different to ballet, although some styles are more influenced than others by balletic choreography and technique. Jazz often incorporates more 'natural' bodily forms, for example, tending away from the 'turned-out' and more formally mannered movements of ballet.

A wide range of popular dance styles come under the jazz dance umbrella including tap dancing and the jitterbug, so it is almost certainly possible to find a style to suit your particular interests and needs. The basic requirement is that the dance must be performed to the rhythm of jazz music.

Jazz dance for fitness

Jazz dance can be a highly energetic form of exercise and so is extremely useful for developing stamina. Its links with ballet also mean it helps to develop similarly high levels of flexibility and muscle strength.

Tap dancing provides a particularly good work-out for the calves and thighs while the jitterbug requires a high level of aerobic fitness. Depending on your energy levels the lifts and swing movements will also demand quite significant muscle strength.

INDEX

Acknowledgments

Carroll & Brown Limited
would like to thank
Charteris Sports Centre
Jennie Crewdson
Holmes Place Gym
Iyengar Yoga Institute
  223a Randolph Avenue
  London W9 1NL
Clare and Diego Luzuraga
Gilda Pacitti
Pilates Centre Ltd

Editorial assistance
Denise Alexander
Jennifer Mussett
Laura Price

Photographic assistants
Lee Mcpherson
Colin Tatham

Picture research
Sandra Schneider
Richard Soar

Photograph sources
8 Louvre, Paris, France/Lauros-Giraudon/Bridgeman Art Library, London
9 (top) Galleria dell'Accademia, Venice/Bridgeman Art Library, London
  (bottom) Sporting Pictures (UK) Ltd
19 The Society of Teachers of the Alexander Technique
20 Rolfing Institute
22 ACE Photo Library
23 (top) Popperfoto
  (bottom) REX Features Ltd
25 Mehau Kulyk/Science Photo Library
26 (left) CNRI/Science Photo Library
  (right) Laguna Design/Science Photo Library
27 (top left) Mary Evans Picture Library/Illustrated London News
  (top right) REX Features Ltd
  (bottom) B&C Alexander
28 (top) AKG London/Erich Lessing
  (bottom) Belvoir Castle, Leicestershire/Bridgeman Art Library, London
29 (left) Rodidnice Lobkowicz Coll, Nelahozeves Castle, Czech Republic/Bridgeman Art Library, London
  (middle) Getty Images
  (right) Mary Evans Picture Library
32 (left) REX Features Ltd
  (right) REX Features Ltd
34 (top) AKG London
  (bottom) ACE Photo Agency/Bill Bachmann
42 Images/The Charles Walker Collection
43 (top left) Jules Selmes
  (top right) The Image Bank
  (bottom left) Jules Selmes
45 (left) The Image Bank
  (middle) The Image Bank
  (right) Getty Images
47 The Image Bank
50 Hellerwork, California
53 Scott Camazine/Science Picture Library
63 Sporting Pictures (UK) Ltd
64 Corbis/UPI
69 Art Directors and TRIP/R. Powers
86 Getty Images
87 Manfred Kage/Science Photo Library
91 Images Colour Library
138 ACE Photo Agency/Kevin Phillips
140 Iyengar Yoga Institute
145 James Davis Travel Photography
147 Musee Conde, Chantilly, France/Lauros Giraudon/Bridgeman Art Library, London
148 Getty Images
154 Art Directors and TRIP/T.Bognar
155 Getty Images
155 James Davis Travel Photography
156 Corbis/UPI

Illustrators
Diane Fisher
John Geary
Connie Jude
Bill Piggins
Natasha Stewart
Halli Verinder
Angela Wood

Hair and make-up
Bettina Graham
Kim Menzies

Index
Jennifer Mussett